REVERSING INFLAMMATION

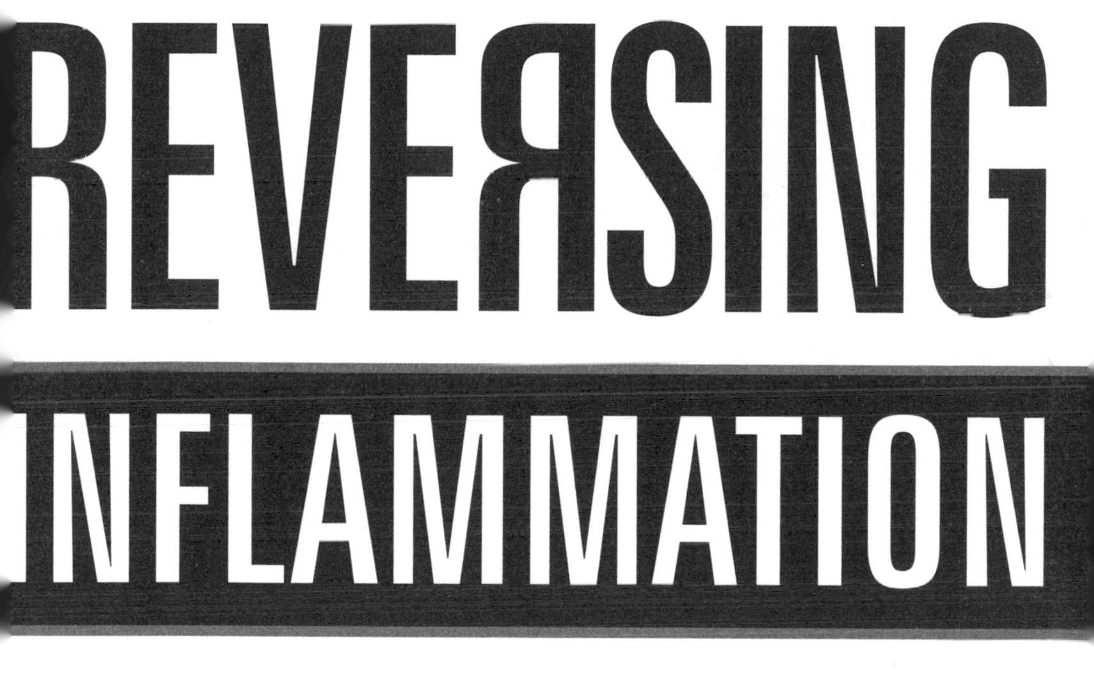

DON COLBERT, MD

SILOAM

Most Charisma House Book Group products are available at special quantity discounts for bulk purchase for sales promotions, premiums, fund-raising, and educational needs. For details, write Charisma House Book Group, 600 Rinehart Road, Lake Mary, Florida 32746, or telephone (407) 333-0600.

Reversing Inflammation by Don Colbert, MD
Published by Siloam
Charisma Media/Charisma House Book Group
600 Rinehart Road
Lake Mary, Florida 32746
www.charismahouse.com

Cover design by Lisa Rae McClure
Design Director: Justin Evans

Visit the author's website at www.drcolbert.com.

Library of Congress Cataloging-in-Publication Data

Colbert, Don.
Reversing inflammation : prevent disease, slow aging, and super-charge your weight loss / Don Colbert, MD.
pages cm
Summary: "Inflammation is an important part of the immune system.

However, problems arise when this reaction becomes systemic and unchecked over a period of time. This book walks the reader through the process of building a healthy lifestyle that can combat the negative effects of inflammation"-- Provided by publisher.
Includes bibliographical references and index.
ISBN 978-1-62998-035-5 (paperback) -- ISBN 978-1-62998-038-6 (e-book)
1. Inflammation--Popular works. 2. Inflammation--Treatment--Popular works. 3. Inflammation--Diet therapy--Popular works. I. Title.
RB131.C65 2015
616'.0473--dc23
2014043984

Portions of this book were previously published by Siloam as *The New Bible Cure for High Blood Pressure*, ISBN 978-1-61638-615-3, copyright © 2013; *The New Bible Cure for Weight Loss*, ISBN 978-1-61638-616-0, copyright © 2013; *Reversing Diabetes*, ISBN 978-1-61638-598-9, copyright © 2012; *Dr. Colbert's "I Can Do This" Diet*, ISBN 978-1-61638-267-4, copyright © 2010; *The New Bible Cure for Heart Disease*, ISBN 978-1-59979-869-1, copyright © 2010; *The New Bible Cure for Diabetes*, ISBN 978-1-59979-759-5, copyright © 2009; *The Bible Cure for Autoimmune Diseases*, ISBN 978-0-88419-939-7, copyright © 2004; and *The Bible Cure for Arthritis*, ISBN 978-0-88419-649-5, copyright © 1999.

stories of individuals described in this book to individuals known to readers is purely coincidental.

The statements in this book about consumable products or food have not been evaluated by the Food and Drug Administration. The recipes in this book are to be followed exactly as written. The publisher is not responsible for your specific health or allergy needs that may require medical supervision. The publisher is not responsible for any adverse reactions to the consumption of food or products that have been suggested in this book.

15 16 17 18 19 — 987654321
Printed in the United States of America

CONTENTS

Introduction

WHAT IS INFLAMMATION?

After the first decade of the new millennium the American Southwest could have been renamed the Burning Region. Of more than two dozen major wildfires in North America since 2002, nearly 60 percent occurred in such states as California, Nevada, New Mexico, and Arizona.

It started with the largest fire in Sequoia National Forest history in California in 2002. Other blazes in the Southwest followed that killed people, burned millions of acres, destroyed thousands of homes, and caused billions of dollars' worth of damage. When the largest fire in Arizona's history struck in the summer of 2011, it destroyed more than 700 square miles of land and spread into New Mexico.[1]

Every fall it seems some state in this region is bracing for another string of wildfires, hoping the winds won't blow too hard and cause the fires to spread. I remember flying over California in the autumn of 2007. I looked out my window and saw separate fires smoldering almost everywhere. It is a moment I would describe as a Salvador Dali painting come to life.

This same surreal picture describes the blazes that are rampantly burning inside many Americans today. However, while the southwestern fires hold the nation's attention for weeks on end, most of us are completely unaware of what is aflame. Sadly this fire—known as *systemic inflammation*—continues to wreak havoc on millions of people, leading many toward obesity, disease, and potentially death.

Inflammation: The Good and the Bad

Inflammation actually means "fire inside," because inflamed areas often feel as if they are burning from within. Inflammation is the redness, swelling, pain, and heat that occur in an area of the body as a consequence of infection, injury, or a foreign object such as a splinter. For example, if you have strep tonsillitis, your tonsils are infected with a strep bacterium, and they are generally swollen, red, and very painful. A sprained ankle is simply inflammation in the ankle, and the ankle is usually red, swollen, painful, and warm. A splinter that is embedded in your skin may eventually form an abscess or boil that is red, swollen, warm, and painful.

This is the good side of inflammation—the healing side. Acute inflammation is meant to save your life or speed up healing by sending white blood cells to the area that is inflamed in order to fight the infection, splint the injury, or wall off the inflammation, which occurs in an abscess. It is an important component of the immune system, essential for the healing process as a programmed response and necessary for fighting infections and repairing damaged tissues.

Acute inflammation on the molecular level is similar to a war. First, your immune system recognizes an invader such as an infection or injury and sends troops in the form of white blood cells to the area being attacked by using chemical signals. Similar to troops going into battle, these white blood cells receive instructions to defend the area that is injured or under attack. The white blood cells then swarm the injured area and secrete different chemical "weapons" in order to eradicate the infection. Now you are beginning to visualize the good side of inflammation—its role in fighting invaders such as bacteria and viruses and eliminating them from the body.

Now let's look at the dark side of inflammation. Realize that the same inflammation that can save your life in the short term can also kill you if inflammation becomes chronic. Problems arise when this inflammatory reaction becomes systemic and goes unchecked for months or years. When this happens, the same chemicals used for healing can cause weight gain and eventually trigger a host of deadly diseases.

JUST SAY NO

Aspirin and ibuprofen may seem like quick, easy, and affordable solutions for reducing inflammation. The same is true for various steroids (prednisone, cortisone, and Medrol) and nonsteroidal anti-inflammatory drugs (NSAIDs). However, keep in mind that when used long term, all of these come with a potentially serious cost, such as the increased likelihood of heart attacks, stroke, and other ailments.

Localized inflammation is easy to spot and feel. Its signs include swelling, redness, warmth, and pain. When the body triggers this healing response, you feel the pain of a strained muscle, a sprain, tendonitis, or bursitis. However, since systemic inflammation does not normally provide these symptoms, it goes unrecognized. Worse, when it is finally diagnosed, doctors and patients often dismiss it as a mere sign of aging or obesity. Unfortunately this oversight often leads to further weight gain and disease.

While chronic inflammation is a symptom of virtually every disease, it also aggravates the disease. Unremitting inflammation brings exposure to inflammatory cytokines, which are destructive, cell-signaling chemicals that contribute to most degenerative diseases. Among them are atherosclerosis, heart disease, cancer, arthritis, metabolic syndrome, Alzheimer's disease, allergies, asthma, ulcerative colitis, Crohn's disease, hepatitis, celiac disease, and diabetes.

You'll notice that almost all of these diseases are linked to obesity. Essentially, as Americans get fatter, chronic systemic inflammation increases and leads to many of these diseases. It also causes our bodies to age rapidly, including developing wrinkles. One of the primary ways to defeat inflammation, then, is through weight loss and a healthy lifestyle.

The good news is, there is much you can do to change the course of your health. As you learn about inflammation, understand its causes, and take the practical, positive steps detailed in this book, you will reverse inflammation in your body and discover the abundant life promised by Jesus when He said, "I have come that they may have life, and that they may have it more abundantly" (John 10:10). In this book you will learn how to fight chronic inflammation—especially inflammation related to inflammation-specific ailments such as heart disease, diabetes, arthritis, Crohn's disease, and a few others. What's more, you will learn how to battle its insidious presence with a very doable, natural plan: through diet, exercise, and overall nutrition.

Now is the time to run to the battle with fresh confidence, renewed determination, and the wonderful knowledge that God is real, alive, and more powerful than any sickness or disease. Each chapter ends with action steps for you to take to incorporate what you are learning. Record your answers in your food journal—or a notebook. It is my prayer that the suggestions and guidelines outlined in this book will help improve your health, nutritional habits, and fitness practices. This combination will bring wholeness to your life. I pray that they will deepen your fellowship with God and strengthen your ability to worship and serve Him.

Section I

LEARN THE LANDSCAPE

Chapter 1

HEART DISEASE

Have you ever considered the marvelous design and operation of your cardiovascular system? It's the body's amazing superhighway. The large arteries within it are much like interstate expressways, and the smaller arteries are like streets and side streets. The primary function of the circulatory system is to deliver oxygen and nutrients to all the cells in your body and to remove cellular debris and waste.

Each day your heart beats approximately 100,000 times, pushing about 2,000 gallons of blood through the 60,000 miles of blood vessels in your body, which include arteries, veins, and capillaries.[1] Despite this incredible distance, blood circulates throughout your entire system about once a minute.[2] Thus your heart will beat more than 2.5 billion times if you live an average lifespan, and it will pump more than 1 million barrels of blood.[3] This superhighway system is truly wonderful.

Wouldn't it be a good idea to keep this blood vessel superhighway free of traffic jams?

Building a Deadly Backup

Yes, we might think of heart problems in terms of traffic flow—and a traffic jam. The worst contributor to a potentially deadly backup is a condition called *atherosclerosis*, which attacks the heart's blood vessels. The arteries that supply the heart with blood and nourishment are the coronary arteries. These are the most stressed arteries of the body because they're squeezed flat from the pumping action of the heart.

Atherosclerosis is the hardening of these arteries most commonly due to excessive amounts of plaque. This plaque contains cholesterol, calcium, white blood cells, collagen, elastin, platelets, and other materials. You could compare plaque to a buildup of debris in a pipe. As the plaque builds up in the arteries, blood flow is eventually decreased to vital organs, including the heart and brain. This buildup can lead to an interruption of blood flow to an artery in the brain, which causes a stroke. When blood flow is interrupted in a coronary artery, a heart attack occurs.

Here's the fender-bender in this traffic jam. In the United States more than 780,000 people a year die from disease related to the cardiovascular system. Nearly another 130,000 die from strokes, which are the equivalent of a "heart attack of the brain."[4] While the good news is that these numbers are on the decrease, the bad news is that cardiovascular disease is still the leading cause of death in the United States.

Instead of becoming one of these statistics, you can take positive steps naturally and spiritually to beat heart disease. The risk of heart attacks can still be greatly lessened through dietary and lifestyle changes. In fact, cardiovascular disease is one of the most treatable and preventable of all afflictions, despite the fact that it causes more than one in three of all deaths in the United States every year.[5] That means you can fight back, overcome, and win the battle. Through lifestyle changes, good nutrition, prayer, and Scripture reading, you can respond in confident hope to this disease.

The initial symptoms and warning signs of heart disease are not a death sentence, but they are a life warning. Change is required. Positive steps must be taken. The way you live and eat cannot remain the same if you want to have a healthy and strong heart.

Freeing Up the Traffic

If atherosclerosis is the cause of a traffic jam in the blood flow, you'll be happy to know that forces are at work in your body to free up the traffic jam. I can explain this best by breaking the process into two parts—(1) the problem of free radicals and (2) the problem of inflammation, which is our main focus in this book—to free you from the constraints and impact of inflammation on your health.

DID YOU KNOW...?

Plaque in the coronary artery usually starts developing in our teens. During the Korean War when soldiers died in battle at an average age of twenty-two, they were autopsied, and three-quarters of them had plaque in their coronary arteries, many of whom had advanced atherosclerotic plaque. A study was done on three thousand bodies age fourteen to thirty-five who were autopsied after death from auto accident, homicide, or suicide. Of those autopsied, 20 to 25 percent had a major lesion in their coronary arteries.[6]

The problem: oxidative stress

First, though, let's discuss the problem of free radicals. A free radical isn't a terrorist trying to bomb our embassy; rather, it's a defective molecule that sends out molecular shrapnel, damaging the coronary arteries and other cells in our bodies.

To envision this problem, think about the oxidation process. Burn wood in a fireplace, and smoke is a by-product. Likewise, when you metabolize food into energy, oxygen oxidizes (or burns) the food in order to produce energy. This process does not create smoke like burning wood in a fireplace, but it does produce dangerous by-products known as *free radicals*. These are molecules that have electrons roaming free to do damage in other cells. Isn't it ironic that breathing oxygen is critical for life and that oxygen usage by the cells is our bodies' greatest source of free radicals?

With regard to heart disease, the problem is that free radicals wreak havoc on the linings of arteries. You see, the lining of the coronary arteries is comprised of very sensitive cells that can easily sustain damage by free radicals produced from oxygen free radicals, cigarette smoke, hypertension, excessive stress, high cholesterol, high lipoprotein(a), elevated homocysteine, and other risk factors. Oxidation is a normal biochemical process in the body. However, sometimes excessive amounts of free radicals are produced, or we have inadequate antioxidant protection. This oxidative stress can damage healthy cells and tissues, including the lining of the arteries or endothelium. When LDL cholesterol is oxidized, it is especially damaging to the arterial lining and is associated with plaque formation.

So, free radicals are the enemies of our blood vessels and of our bodies' cells in general. Some estimates calculate that the cells in our bodies may sustain over ten thousand hits from free radicals each day, especially if we have inadequate antioxidants.

CHOLESTEROL ISN'T THE CULPRIT

Current research is finding that LDL and total cholesterol levels alone are not the best indicators of whether or not heart attacks will happen. Approximately half the time cardiac arrest is the first symptom of cardiovascular disease someone will experience, and doctors estimate that about 50 percent of those with normal cholesterol levels will still have heart attacks or strokes. While those with high LDL and total cholesterol are three times more likely than those with low levels to experience heart attacks or strokes, there are far too many with "acceptable" levels who have heart attacks every day.[7] Approximately half the patients who suffer heart attacks have normal cholesterol levels. Many individuals think that because their cholesterol is normal or low, they are protected against cardiovascular disease. How wrong they are! Hosea 4:6 says, "My people are destroyed for lack of knowledge" (KJV).

The solution: antioxidants

The heart is the hardest-working organ in the body. Since the coronary arteries sustain more wear and tear than other arteries, they also need to be constantly repaired. God's cure in winning the battle against heart disease includes a powerful weapon against free radicals—antioxidants. They're amazing substances that slow oxidation and block or repair free-radical reactions in our bodies. Antioxidants are extremely important in preventing heart disease due to their blocking and repairing functions.

Millions of microscopic cracks and damaged areas may occur inside the artery walls from oxidative damage. When the body does not have adequate amounts of antioxidants, especially glutathione and vitamins C and E, in order to repair the lining of damaged blood vessels, it will be more prone to forming plaque in the arteries. This, along with chronic inflammation, which we'll discuss next, forms fatty streaks in the blood vessels and leads to plaque formation. However, adequate amounts of antioxidants such as glutathione, vitamins C and E, bioflavonoids, pine bark and grape seed extract, resveratrol, pomegranate juice, and berries such as blueberries, blackberries, raspberries, and strawberries may help prevent these cracks from occurring in the first place. (See appendix.)

Picture it this way: Imagine repairing a house after a tornado has partially damaged the roof and damaged the walls. If you didn't have the money to repair the roof and walls properly and merely patched them with the inexpensive materials at hand, the next storm might well destroy your dwelling for good.

Likewise if you have inadequate antioxidants in your diet and you are damaging your blood vessels with smoking, high blood pressure, or a fatty diet, areas of your blood vessels will usually become chronically inflamed and attract *monocytes* (white blood cells), which are transformed into *macrophages*, another type of white blood cell. These macrophages are super garbage collectors that gobble up oxidized cholesterol and cellular debris and eventually form fatty streaks and, later, fatty plaque.

However, antioxidant vitamins help to prevent or repair the lining of the blood vessels that are damaged and to halt or diminish the destructive inflammatory response. Without adequate antioxidants, more plaque is formed. If this continues over decades, the fatty plaque builds up in your blood vessels, creating atherosclerosis, which can eventually lead to a heart attack. This certainly isn't God's will for you!

For a healthy heart don't forget your citrus fruit and vitamin C. Vitamin C is a very important antioxidant for repairing damage to the coronary arteries. It helps to increase the production of collagen and elastin, both of which add stability to your blood vessels. Collagen produced without vitamin C is weaker and causes blood vessels to become fragile. Scurvy results from an extremely depleted supply of vitamin C reserves in the body. This condition causes a gradual breakdown of collagen, leading to a breakdown in blood vessels, resulting in internal hemorrhaging.

FAST FACT

While many animals can create their own vitamin C, people cannot. We must replenish it daily through our diet. Unfortunately much of our food is so processed that very little vitamin C remains in our foods. Citrus fruit is a major source of vitamin C, but while most of us may have enough vitamin C to prevent scurvy, we don't have enough to win the war against arteriosclerosis.

Inflammation: The Root Cause of Heart Disease

Heart disease is hidden in more than half of all adults over the age of thirty-five. That is more than half of your family and friends. Many think that because their cholesterol is normal, they are protected against heart disease, but science is finding that keeping our arteries healthy is about much more than just cholesterol levels. About half of the people who have heart attacks have normal cholesterol levels. The root cause of heart disease is not high cholesterol but inflammation.

Your coronary arteries are composed of three layers. Most think of arteries and blood vessels as simple, supple tubes, but in reality they are dynamic muscular structures that expand and contract to aid in circulation and keep blood pressure stable. The outer layer is the adventitia. The middle layer is made of smooth muscle, which enables the arteries to dilate and constrict and is called the medial layer. The inner layer, called the intima or endothelium, is smooth like Teflon and is a very thin layer only one cell thick.

As we age, areas of the smooth and slick endothelium lining of the arteries eventually become injured by various factors, including high blood pressure, oxidation of LDL cholesterol, cigarette smoke, free radicals, elevated homocysteine levels, elevated C-reactive protein (CRP) levels, elevated blood sugar and insulin levels, bad fats, poor diet, toxic chemicals and metals, and more. These single or combined insults to areas of the coronary arteries kindle inflammation, which is what leads to atherosclerosis.

DID YOU KNOW...?

A simple warning sign of heart disease is a diagonal crease in the earlobes. If you have creases in the earlobes, there is a strong probability you have significant atherosclerosis in your coronary arteries.[8] Also, according to a Harvard study, men who are losing the hair on the crown of their heads have up to a 34 percent greater risk of having cardiovascular problems.[9]

The presence of chemicals associated with inflammation called *cytokines* causes the inner layer of the arteries to become more like Velcro rather than Teflon. In areas of the coronary arteries that have been damaged by high blood pressure, cigarette smoke, or other factors, the presence of these inflammatory cytokines attracts a type of white blood cell called *monocytes*, as I mentioned above.

These monocytes eventually transform into *macrophages*, which are even more powerful than the monocytes. Macrophages gobble up dead cells as well as cellular garbage, including oxidized cholesterol. These macrophages eat and eat, literally stuffing themselves with oxidized cholesterol and cellular garbage as they continue to grow larger and larger.

When chronic inflammation is present, the macrophages continue to eat and may grow so large that they appear like foam and are called *foam cells*. As inflammation continues, the macrophages continue to eat until they eventually eat themselves to death. When they die, their contents are spilled in the arterial wall and appear as a fatty yellow streak inside the artery. Because of this, researchers are beginning to realize treating heart disease may be more about controlling chronic inflammation than about simply lowering cholesterol levels in the bloodstream.

However, if you quench the fire of inflammation, your arteries will attempt to heal themselves by forming a fibrous cap. A fibrous cap is called stable plaque and is much less likely to rupture than unstable plaque. The fibrous cap consists of scar tissue and will typically remain stable as long as the inflammation is controlled. In addition to this, there is good evidence that by quenching chronic inflammation and modifying certain risk factors, you may be able to stabilize the plaque and sometimes actually reverse atherosclerosis.

If inflammation is not stopped and chronic inflammation continues unabated, the fatty streak will continue to grow into fatty plaque. As these foam cells die and release their fatty contents, the plaque forms a fatty core, which is a soft yellow liquid similar in consistency to liquid margarine. As this process continues, the fatty core will keep expanding as more and more macrophages continue to eat and eat the oxidized cholesterol and cellular garbage and continue to grow and eventually die. Ultimately, if this inflammatory process is not stopped, your body's own immune system may actually kill you through mechanisms involving chronic inflammation.

Chronic inflammation may eventually cause the fibrous cap to rupture, similar to popping a large pimple. The fatty, liquid margarine–like material will ooze out of the plaque. Immediately platelets will stick to the oozing fatty material like a swarm of flies to flypaper, and a blood clot forms. As this blood clot blocks the flow of blood, it cuts off vital oxygen and nutrients and causes a heart attack or stroke, depending on which artery it occurs in. If it occurs in a coronary artery, a heart attack occurs. If it occurs in a cerebral or carotid artery, a stroke occurs. Approximately 80 percent of heart attacks are a result of ruptured plaque.[10]

If you are lucky enough to reach the hospital in time, the doctor will quickly give you a clot-busting drug or insert a stent to open the blocked artery. A clot-busting drug will dissolve the clot, allowing the blood to flow again to the heart, but it does not dissolve the plaque. Individuals typically do not accumulate plaque in just one or two areas but in dozens of areas. Each area may rupture, and just one rupture can cause a heart attack. Also, a plaque buildup may cause only a 20 percent blockage, but even that small an area of plaque can still rupture and cause a heart attack.

This is the dark side of inflammation, which is at the root of most heart disease. There is, however, very good news: we can quench the fires of chronic inflammation. Consuming a diet that is anti-inflammatory as well as taking specific antioxidants and nutrients can effectively quench the fires of inflammation and prevent—and in many cases even reverse—cardiovascular disease. We will explore these life-producing changes later in this book.

DR. COLBERT APPROVED—TEST YOUR INFLAMMATION LEVEL

Chronic inflammation can be detected by a simple blood test. We now have a blood test that measures the level of C-reactive protein (CRP) that detects the chronic inflammation that contributes to coronary artery disease.[11]

C-reactive protein is both a marker of inflammation and a promoter of inflammation. Elevated CRP blood levels create a constant environment prone to inflammation within your entire body. When CRP levels are high, every cell in your body is vulnerable to the damaging effects of inflammation. When this chronic inflammation occurs in the blood vessels, it usually causes the atherosclerosis, which is the first step toward having a heart attack and stroke. This is why in 2003 the American Heart Association (AHA) and the Centers for Disease Control and Prevention (CDC) started recommending adding CRP blood tests to regular annual checkups.

Numerous recent studies have shown that CRP is likely a better predictor of heart attack and stroke risk than traditional cholesterol tests alone. Those with elevated CRP levels but acceptable cholesterol levels are more likely to have heart attacks or strokes than those with high cholesterol but low CRP. Also, those with high CRP levels are less likely to survive when a heart attack or stroke does occur. I think we will be seeing more in the media in the coming years about testing CRP levels as an important means of detecting chronic cardiovascular risk.

CRP is produced in many cells of the body in response to the presence of the cytokines that promote inflammation. C-reactive protein is mainly produced by fat cells, especially belly fat, and the liver in response to excess interleukin-6—a cytokine. CRP is released by abdominal fat and then is dumped directly into the liver. As a result, those who are overweight or obese, especially those who have abdominal fat, often have significantly higher levels of CRP in their bloodstreams than do lean people.

CRP RANGES FOR MEN AND WOMEN

Men CRP (mg/L)	Relative Risk For:	
	Future MI (heart attack)	Future Stroke
>2.11	2.9	1.9
1.15–2.10	2.6	1.9
0.56–1.14	1.7	1.7
<0.55	1.0	1.0

Women CRP (mg/L)	Relative Risk for Future MI or Stroke
>7.3	5.5
3.8–7.3	3.5
1.5–3.7	2.7
<1.5	1.0

To reduce CRP levels, you should follow the Mediterranean diet outlined in chapter 10 and avoid foods high in saturated fats and trans fats. You should also avoid fried foods and foods that are high glycemic—or raise the blood sugar rapidly. Sweets, white bread, white rice, and instant potatoes are prime examples of high-glycemic foods. Instead, you can choose to eat foods high in fiber, such as raw almonds, lentils, beans, peas, seeds, nuts, apples, berries, and so forth. Again, eating a Mediterranean diet is one of the simplest ways to lower CRP as well as many other risk factors.

A superantioxidant found in French maritime pine bark or made from combinations of grape seed, pine bark, and red wine extract has been shown to lower CRP levels. Studies have shown oligomeric proanthocyanidins (OPCs) can lower CRP by 50 percent.[12] Most studies have used doses of 120 to 300 mg daily. (See appendix.)

Another way to address CRP levels is by taking daily supplements that include (see appendix):

- Fish oil, pharmaceutical grade (1,000 mg, two to three times a day)

- Coenzyme Q_{10} (ubiquinol) (100–200 mg a day)
- Pine bark extract and grape seed extract, or OPCs (120–300 mg a day)
- Red yeast rice, or LipiControl (1,200 mg, twice a day with food)
- Irvingia extract (150 mg, twice a day)

Better Information Makes for a Better Future

Altogether this may seem overwhelming, but here's the good news. First, cardiovascular disease is totally preventable if we take the proper precautions to quench chronic inflammation. Second, my experience in medicine tells me that no matter what condition your heart is in today, there is hope for health and recovery—yes, even if your parents or grandparents suffered from heart disease. If you'll follow the recommendations in this chapter, as well as the changes to diet, nutrition, and exercise outlined later in this book, you will discover that clogged arteries can often be reversed without surgery.

Healthy lifestyle choices like the anti-inflammatory diet and other recommendations I will be explaining later are the best way to lower risk factors that lead to arterial inflammation. Where most doctors will recommend statin drugs as a solution, I would caution you before following that course. Study after study has shown that lifestyle changes, if combined with a healthy diet and proper nutritional supplements, can have the same or better results than taking a daily statin drug, and without the side effects.

And remember God's Word with regard to everything I'm saying. Health and healing are what the Lord has in mind for you, just as He told the prophet long ago:

> "For I will restore health to you and heal you of your wounds," says the LORD.
>
> —JEREMIAH 30:17

Here's more good news: the number of cardiovascular-related deaths in the United States is declining. Before the turn into this millennium the American Heart Association (AHA) had reported that one in two deaths was related to heart disease. However, according to 2014 AHA statistics, just over one in three deaths in the United States are now related to cardiovascular disease, a category of illnesses that includes high blood pressure, coronary heart disease, heart attack, angina, heart failure, and stroke.[13] In fact, the AHA reports that from 1996 to 2006, the death rate from cardiovascular disease declined by 29 percent.[14]

While the trends reflected by these statistics are encouraging, we can also be optimistic because heart disease is one of the most preventable of all degenerative diseases. Furthermore, we can take great hope in the reality that God is our healer (Exod. 15:26). Nutrition and lifestyle changes are the cornerstones in keeping it at bay. Prayer is a great resource in building our hope and opening our lives up to God's healing power.

Yes, there is hope for this amazing, hardworking superhighway vascular system in your body. It can keep the nutrients flowing for years and years with no roadblocks or breakdowns. So I encourage you to live each day in faith and hope, while taking some important preventive steps right away.

Action Steps

1. What is your experience with heart disease (personal experience, family or friends who have experience)?
2. What fears do you have concerning heart disease in your life?
3. Which of the following antioxidants can you include in your diet to quench free radicals?
   - Citrus fruits
   - Pomegranate juice
   - Berries
   - Vitamin C
   - Bioflavonoids
   - Pine bark and grape seed extract
   - Vitamin E
   - Glutathione-boosting supplements
   - Resveratrol

Chapter 2

WEIGHT GAIN

Before the finger of God touched the oceans with unimaginable creative power, God envisioned you in His heart. He saw you and all you could one day be through the power of His supernatural grace. You are God's masterpiece, designed according to an eternal plan so awesome that it's beyond your ability to comprehend.

Have you ever wondered what He saw in His mind when He created you? What was the perfection of purpose and plan He intended?

Now close your eyes and see yourself. For one moment you have no bondages, no imperfections, no shortcomings. Your body is as lean and healthy as it could possibly be. What do you look like? Is that the person God had in mind?

If you've struggled with weight gain or obesity all of your life, you may not even be able to imagine yourself free of the bondage of unwanted fat. But God can. Don't you think that if God is powerful enough to create you and the entire universe that you see around you, He is also able to help you overcome all of your personal bondages? Of course He is!

Let's look together at the reasons for weight gain that lead to ill health, as well as the role inflammation plays in its development, and then discover the plan for becoming the person you saw or imagined when you closed your eyes. Mixed together with the power of God found in prayer and Scripture, you will discover strength for success that is beyond your own ability to give you the freedom and joy of a healthy, fit, more attractive you!

An Obesity Epidemic

If you have a weight problem, you're not alone. In recent years America has experienced an alarming rise in obesity. Two-thirds of American adults are overweight or obese, and 30 percent of children age eleven or younger are overweight.[1] This should concern everyone, particularly those of us who profess Jesus as Savior and Lord. God revealed His divine will for each of us through the apostle John, who wrote, "Beloved, I pray that you may prosper in all things and be in health, just as your soul prospers" (3 John 2). With obesity at almost epidemic proportions, surely we are missing God's best.

Research tells us that, in the United States, an estimated 300,000 deaths per year are attributed to obesity.[2] Obesity also comes with a fat price tag (pun intended). People considered obese pay $1,429 more (42 percent) in health care costs than normal-weight individuals.[3] And as shocking as all this sounds, no dollar amount can do justice to the real damage being done. Being overweight or obese increases your risk of developing thirty-five major diseases, particularly type 2 diabetes, heart disease, stroke, arthritis, hypertension, acid reflux, sleep apnea, Alzheimer's, infertility, erectile dysfunction, and gallbladder disease—plus more than a dozen forms of cancer.

Besides obesity's physical implications, it carries a social and psychological impact. Obese individuals generally contend with more rejection and prejudice. Often they are overlooked for promotions or not even hired because of physical appearance. Most obese people struggle daily with issues of self-worth and self-image. They feel unattractive and unappreciated and are at an increased risk of depression. Many of us have watched the humiliation an obese person experiences trying to squeeze into an airplane, stadium, or automobile seat that is too small. Maybe you have been that person. If so, you know how obesity can affect the way others treat you and how you treat yourself.

Chances are that if you are struggling with obesity, you may have been waging a war with it all of your life. By now you realize that you need more than a good dieting program. You need power to enforce it. You need the strength it takes to change a lifetime of poor eating habits and the discipline to stay with it. Stop limiting yourself to your own strength. The Bible reveals a better way:

> I can do all things through Christ who strengthens me.
>
> —Philippians 4:13

Gaining new power in your battle against obesity must begin with gaining fresh understanding of the causes for obesity. Instead of looking for the next new-and-improved medication to manage obesity-related disease, you need to get to the root of the problem. It turns out that there are a number of them.

DID YOU KNOW...?

McDonald's feeds an astounding 70 million people a day worldwide, which is more than the entire populations of Canada and Sudan combined![4]

Why We Eat Too Much

Being overweight has many causes. Some are biological. You might be predisposed to obesity through genetics and body metabolism. Some of the causes are psychological. And again, as we'll learn later in this chapter, inflammation can play quite a part in your weight gain. Let's look together at the many causes of weight gain and obesity in society today.

Emotional eating

One reason for your struggle with weight may be that you are emotionally dependent on food for comfort during times of stress, crisis, anxiety, loneliness, and a host of other emotions. If overeating has an emotional component in your life, you probably grew up hearing statements such as the following:

- "Eat something; it will make you feel better."
- "Clean your plate, or you can't leave the table."
- "If you're good, you will get dessert."
- "If you don't eat everything, you will be impolite to the host or hostess."
- "If you stop crying, I'll give you ice cream."

The list of unhealthy childhood motivations can be endless. But whether the causes of your weight problem are genetic or psychological, you are not bound to your past. Today is a new day, filled with fresh hope for an entirely new way of thinking and living. Begin considering what lifestyle factors might be contributing to your situation.

DR. COLBERT APPROVED—DO IT SMART

One of the most important keys to losing weight is establishing attainable goals rather than ones that will leave you frustrated, angry, and most likely gaining weight. That's why virtually every physician says that when starting a diet, aim for a goal of losing no more than 10 to 15 percent of your total body weight. Once you've reached that, set a new goal—but don't jump the gun. While you can dream big (or in this case small), remember that traveling on the road to weight loss happens one step at a time.

A sedentary lifestyle

Another cause of obesity is the increasingly sedentary lifestyle in our society. In an agricultural or industrial culture, hard work gives people plenty of exercise during the day. In our corporate, technological culture we sit more at desks and in meetings. And the problem doesn't just plague adults. Too many children no longer play sports and participate in outdoor activities. Instead they get entranced by video games, smartphones, text messages, social networking, online media, TV, and movies. Combined with their favorite fast food, reducing exercise to a flick of the finger on a remote control spells ever-increasing weight gain.

Excessive stress

The excessive stress that most adults and many children labor under also contributes to our expanding waistlines. Stress increases cortisol levels. As a result, many are developing toxic belly fat, thereby increasing their risk for incurring diabetes and other diseases. Long-term stress eventually depletes stress hormones as well as neurotransmitters. This often helps unleash ravenous appetites, plus addictions to sugar and carbohydrates. It's like a nightmarish vortex, each bad habit working to ensnare sufferers in a downward spiral to poor health and disease.

Too much refined sugar and starch

I believe one of the most important reasons for our epidemic of obesity is our high intake of both refined sugars and starches. The standard American diet is full of empty carbohydrates, sugars, fats, excessive proteins, and calories, and it is low in nutrient content. This diet literally causes us to lose nutrients such as chromium, which is crucial in regulating glucose levels in our blood.

The average person consumes 130 pounds of refined sugar per year.[5] These sugars are sometimes hidden in foods we think are good for us. Take a look at how most of our bread is made. First the outer shell of the grain of wheat is removed. This is the bran or the fiber portion of the grain. The germ of the wheat is then removed; the germ contains the essential fats and vitamin E. These are removed to affect the shelf life of the bread. What is left over is the endosperm, which is the starch of the grain. This is then ground into a very fine powder. The powder of the grain, however, is not white, so it is then bleached with a bleaching agent.

With both the bran and the wheat germ no longer present, and after the bleaching process, very few vitamins remain. Therefore, man-made vitamins are then added back, along with sugar, salt, partially hydrogenated fats, and preservatives. White bread is very constipating because it contains no fiber. Also, since it is highly processed when it is consumed, it is rapidly broken down into sugars, and this then causes high amounts of insulin to be secreted, putting a strain on the pancreas and programming our body to store fat.

A WORD ABOUT WHEAT

The problem with breads, pastas, cereals, and other starches may not be limited to the refining process they undergo. The wheat itself may be the real culprit. Renowned cardiologist William Davis, MD, believes foods made with or containing wheat are the number one reason Americans are fat and suffering from diabetes. Modern wheat strains have been hybridized, crossbred, and genetically altered by agricultural scientists in order to increase crop production.[6] As a result, modern strains of wheat have a higher quantity of genes for gluten proteins that are associated with celiac disease.[7] Modern wheat also contains a starch called amylopectin A, which raises blood sugar levels more than virtually any other carbohydrate.[8]

In addition, wheat is an appetite stimulant, making you want more and more food.[9] It's also considered addictive. Approximately 30 percent of all people who stop eating wheat products experience withdrawal symptoms such as extreme fatigue, mental fog, irritability, inability to function at work, and depression.[10] The addictive nature of wheat, coupled with the fact that it triggers exaggerated blood sugar and insulin responses, sets your body up to pack on the pounds.

I believe that increased consumption of white bread, sugar, processed cereals, and pasta is largely responsible for our epidemic of diabetes, high cholesterol, heart disease, and obesity. In centuries past these refined breads and sugars were given mainly to extremely rich and royal families. This is why many of the wealthy in those days were obese and suffered from diabetes and gout. When we reach the latter part of this book, we will look at specific foods and how they affect our body's function—and what we should eat instead.

FAST FACTS

- Obesity increases your risk of developing the following cancers: esophageal, thyroid, colon, kidney, prostate, endometrial, gallbladder, rectal, breast, pancreatic, leukemia, multiple myeloma, malignant melanoma, and non-Hodgkin's lymphoma [11]
- Being overweight increases your risk of having GERD (acid reflux) symptoms by 50 percent; being obese doubles your chances.[12]
- Excess weight is also commonly known to cause sleep apnea and hypertension (high blood pressure). In fact, 75 percent of all cases of hypertension in the United States is attributed to obesity.[13]

How Fat Is Obese?

Obesity is defined as a body mass index (BMI) of 30 or more. Body mass index is a formula that uses your weight and height to determine if your weight is normal, overweight, or obese. A BMI of 19–24.9 is healthy, a BMI of 25–29.9 is overweight, and a BMI of 30 or more is obese.

However, I hold more stock in body fat percentage than I do the body mass index reading. The reason is simple: accuracy. BMI uses only height and weight to judge how overweight or obese a person is. For example, a twenty-three-year-old professional football player and a fifty-six-year-old executive may both be 5 feet 10 inches tall and weigh 220 pounds. This gives both men a BMI of approximately 35, which is considered obese.

In reality, however, the football player can have a 32-inch waist and a remarkable 6 percent body fat; the executive can have a 44-inch waist and 33 percent body fat. That is an astounding 27 percent differential in body fat percentage alone, which the BMI doesn't take into account.

Although many physicians simply use BMI to determine if a person is overweight or obese, I strongly believe more accurate assessments come from using body fat percentage and waist measurements. However, because it is a helpful tool to measure your weight loss goals, I have included the following chart to help you determine your BMI and which category—normal, overweight, or obese—you are in.

CRP RANGES FOR MEN AND WOMEN

Men CRP (mg/L)	Relative Risk For:	
	Future MI (heart attack)	Future Stroke
>2.11	2.9	1.9
1.15–2.10	2.6	1.9
0.56–1.14	1.7	1.7
<0.55	1.0	1.0

Women CRP (mg/L)	Relative Risk for Future MI or Stroke
>7.3	5.5
3.8–7.3	3.5
1.5–3.7	2.7
<1.5	1.0

Body Fat Percentage

While I see waist size as the most important measurement for establishing weight-loss goals, this does not mean that you can't or shouldn't take other types of measurements—beyond those you can take with a tape measure. Part of the time with patients during their goal-setting stage I spend getting a body fat percentage. I do an initial measurement and then take one a month until they reach their goal.

There are many ways to measure body fat percentage, including bioimpedance analysis, underwater weighing, and using skinfold calipers. Whatever the method, you need to have your body fat percentage measured the same way each time. Consistency is the key, since the percentage can fluctuate dramatically with inaccurate measurements.

DR. COLBERT APPROVED—MEASURING TOOLS

Although skin calipers are the easiest devices for measuring body fat percentage, they can also be the most inaccurate. For a more precise (albeit it sometimes expensive) measurement, try:

- Underwater weighing: Fat floats, while lean tissue sinks—making it easy for specialized hydrostatic weighing equipment to get a highly accurate read on how much fat you're actually carrying.
- Dual X-Ray Absorptiometry (DEXA) scan: Using low-level X-rays, this machine takes into consideration your bone mass and muscle mass to calculate your body fat percentage.
- The Bod Pod: A highly accurate (but again expensive) machine that measures how much air you displace.
- Bioelectrical impedance: Less expensive than the other high-tech tools but pricier (and more precise) than a skin caliper, this method measures the speed of an electrical current as it passes through your body. Unfortunately numerous variables (e.g., full stomach, recent exercise) can sway your results.[14]

Finding your ideal body fat percentage involves two main factors: sex and age. According to the American Council on Exercise, a body fat percentage greater than 26 percent in men and greater than 32 percent in women is considered obese. A healthy percent body fat in women is 25–31 percent, and in men it is 18–25 percent. Initially, obese men should aim for a reading of less than 25 percent, while obese women should shoot for less than 32 percent. Eventually aim for a percent body fat in the healthy range.

However, remember that body fat ranks second to your initial focus to reduce your waist measurement. Don't worry; you will find that body fat percentage will naturally decrease along with your waist measurement. Also, women should remember—because of their hormones—that they will have a higher body fat percentage than men. Female hormones cause distribution of fat in the breasts, hips, thighs, and buttocks. A typical woman should have between 7 and 10 percent more body fat than the average man. Many health clubs, nutritionists, and physicians have the equipment to measure your percentage of body fat. Once you have this initial number, log it in your food journal and get it checked each month.

However, don't get too hung up on body fat or other measurements, such as your BMI reading. Focus on one thing and one thing only: waist measurement. Yes, it's that simple. You really do not need a scale or any other fancy tools—just a tape measure.

A Matter of Weight

For some dieters the idea of not looking at a scale every day sounds foreign. Others feel strange if they don't check at least once a week. Yet after helping thousands of individuals lose weight for good, I have seen how most people do better when they either pack up their scale or get rid of it entirely. The reason is almost purely psychological. When dieters lose the wrong type of weight, such as water weight or muscle weight, their skin may sag or wrinkle, their cheeks and eyes may appear hollow, and their muscle mass may melt away. In the meantime, their metabolic rate decreases, their weight plateaus, and they wind up discouraged because each time they hit the scale, the numbers are still the same. Most often these are the people who quit and regain weight.

Don't get me wrong—weight is important. That is why I always get an initial weight for every patient. Still, because of our weight-obsessed culture, the numbers on a scale can easily become the only measure of success. Though it is tempting to monitor your progress this way, it is not a reliable indicator of fat loss. And losing belly fat should be your primary concern. Avoid the potential depression, guilt, shame, or hopelessness by temporarily putting your scale away. Rely more on an old-fashioned tape measure, a pair of old jeans, a food journal, and a monthly body fat percentage measurement while committing to a monthly weigh-in.

Also, weigh yourself on the same day of each month, and make sure you are fully disrobed. If you are a woman, keep in mind that your weight will fluctuate, based on hormonal fluctuations and your menstrual cycle. So do not get discouraged when this occurs.

Once you reach your goal weight, I then recommend that you weigh yourself daily. That is the only time that I recommend this, since this is the best way to maintain your weight loss.

FIVE "NON-DIGIT" WAYS TO MEASURE WEIGHT LOSS

1. Overall attitude
2. Energy level
3. Fit of clothes
4. Friendly comments and compliments
5. Feeling of taking up less space

What Fruit Are You?

It's not only important to understand *if* you're overweight, but you should also be aware of *how* you're overweight. Let me explain.

Apple-shaped

Where is your body's excess fat located? Do you have belly fat with love handles? If you are a person with abdominal obesity, or central obesity, you are considered "apple-shaped."

If you are apple-shaped, you are much more likely to develop high blood pressure, diabetes, strokes, and coronary artery disease. The reason is this: when your fat is mainly in your abdomen, it is associated with elevated levels of C-reactive protein. As we already discussed in chapter 2, CRP is a marker and a promoter of inflammation, which is the root cause of atherosclerosis or plaque buildup.

Here's how you can determine if you have an apple shape. Simply measure the narrowest area around your waist at the level of your navel and the widest area around your hips. Divide the measurement of your waist by the measurement of your hips. If this number is greater than 0.95 in men or greater than 0.8 in women, then you have an apple shape.

Many patients with apple-shaped obesity also tend to be insulin resistant. When you are insulin resistant, your cells do not properly respond to insulin. As you eat a meal with a lot of sugars or processed, refined starches, these sugars and starches break down into glucose, which is then absorbed into the bloodstream. Glucose triggers the pancreas to secrete insulin. Insulin then causes glucose and other nutrients to be delivered into the cells. As glucose enters the cells, the glucose levels in the blood fall, which then signals the pancreas to stop producing insulin.

But in many obese patients these insulin receptors in the cells do not work properly. Therefore sufficient amounts of glucose and nutrients do not reach the cells, which causes the glucose to remain in the blood. The high levels of blood glucose trigger the pancreas to continue secreting insulin. Now you have high levels of both glucose and insulin. Over time this situation usually leads to type 2 diabetes, which we will discuss in greater detail in the next chapter. As insulin levels and blood sugars rise, they usually lead to elevated cholesterol and triglyceride levels, which eventually accumulate in the arteries as plaque.

Pear-shaped

If your extra fat is stored in your thighs, hips, and buttocks, you are "pear-shaped." This body shape is not nearly as dangerous as apple-shaped obesity.

The Worst Kind of Fat

You may not like the number on your scale, but that figure does not tell the whole story regarding your overall health. Researchers are finding that one of the greatest indicators of potential health problems is having a high percentage of belly fat.

The fat that settles in the belly is different from other types of fat in the body. Fatty tissue or fat storage areas, such as belly fat, are active endocrine organs that produce numerous types of hormones, such as resistin (which increases insulin resistance), leptin (which decreases appetite), and adiponectin (which improves insulin sensitivity and helps to lower blood sugar). The more belly fat cells you have, typically the more estrogen, cortisol, and testosterone your body produces. This is one of the reasons obese men typically develop breasts and obese women often grow hair on their faces. Their fat cells are manufacturing more estrogen and testosterone, respectively.

When your fatty tissues spew out all these hormones—most likely raising your estrogen, testosterone, and cortisol levels—and produce tremendous inflammation in your body, the result is weight gain. Your extra toxic belly fat then sets the stage for type 2 diabetes, heart disease, stroke, cancer, and a host of other diseases. That's because belly fat is like a wildfire. It spreads throughout your body and inflames your cardiovascular system, which eventually causes the production of plaque in your arteries and inflammation in the brain. This can even potentially lead to Alzheimer's disease.

The dangers of this toxic belly fat is one reason I encourage you to set a weight-loss goal based on your waistline rather than your body weight. Typically if your waist measurement increases, your blood sugar will increase; if your waist measurement decreases, your blood sugar will decrease. By reducing your waist measurement, you will probably reverse your risk of many diseases. In fact, lowering waist size ranks higher than weight loss.

Although it is helpful to weigh yourself on a regular basis, I want you to start looking at your waistline as a key indicator of weight management. You should measure your waist around your navel (and love handles, if you have them). Initially your waist measurement goal should be 40 inches or less if you're a man and 35 inches or less if you're a woman. But your ultimate goal should be to have a waist measurement that is half your height or less. For example, a 5-foot-10-inch man is 70 inches tall, so his waist around the belly button and love handles should be 35 inches or less.

EXPANDING WAISTS

Over the past four decades the average American male's waist size has gone from 35 inches to 39 (11 percent). Among women it has increased even more, going from 30 inches to 37 (23 percent). According to the National Institutes of Health, nearly 39 percent of men and 60 percent of women are carrying too much belly fat.[15]

The Connection Between Belly Fat and Inflammation

Now, what does inflammation have to do with weight gain? Let's begin by noting that the obesity and inflammation connection is cyclical in nature: obesity causes increased inflammation, and increased inflammation causes more weight gain. This is partially due to fat cells manufacturing various types of inflammatory mediators, including interleukin-6, tumor necrosis factor-alpha, and plasminogen activator inhibitor-1. These all increase inflammation and are associated with atherosclerosis, or hardening of the arteries, which we discussed in the last chapter as triggers for heart disease.

Fat cells also produce the aforementioned cytokines. These are proteins that trigger the production of more inflammatory mediators, such as C-reactive protein. As I mentioned in the last chapter, CRP is just one inflammatory marker that doctors use to measure the body's inflammatory state. If there is inflammation anywhere in the body, CRP typically increases. The CRP level rises in cases of chronic infection and elevated blood sugar (insulin resistance), and in overweight and obese people, especially among those with increased belly fat. Elevated CRP is also associated with an increased risk of both heart attack and stroke.

When the body produces more inflammatory mediators, such as CRP, this in turn sparks chronic systemic inflammation. Essentially the more fat you have (particularly belly fat), the more inflammation you suffer, which triggers the arteries to constrict. We know that inflammation is the root cause of most coronary artery disease or plaque buildup in the arteries that nourish the heart.

Several studies show the parallels between inflammation and fat. One study found that inflammation increased more than 50 percent in obese women whose fat was primarily in their hips and thighs. Among women with abdominal obesity, that number rose to a staggering 400 percent.[16]

Furthermore, every pound of stored fat requires about a mile's worth of blood vessels to sustain itself. In order to exist, fat cells secrete hormone-like substances to increase blood vessel growth. These blood vessels are supposed to nourish and feed accumulated fat. However, when the blood vessel growth cannot keep up with expanding fat, the fat cells become deprived of oxygen. These oxygen-deprived cells then release more inflammatory mediators to trigger more blood vessel growth...and on it goes. The wildfire spreads, made worse when the spark comes from belly fat, the most flammable source.

Other studies underscore the fact that inflammation not only prepares the body for adding additional fat but also even precedes this process. Two studies, the Atherosclerosis Risk in Communities Study and the Healthy Women Study, found higher concentrations of CRP and fibrinogen before weight gain occurred.[17] (Fibrinogen is a protein in the blood that, when elevated, can lead to blood clots or an increased risk of heart attacks and strokes.) Further research from Sweden showed that the higher the number of elevated inflammatory proteins, the greater the chances of weight gain.[18] Prior to these reports experts assumed that obese people had higher levels of inflammatory proteins because of the cytokines their fatty tissues secreted. In other words, doctors thought that obese individuals continued to deal with greater inflammation because they were obese. Instead, these studies proved the other way was equally true: the higher the inflammatory proteins, the greater the odds of weight gain.

Without a doubt, fat deposited in the abdominal area leads to the greatest amount of inflammation. Conversely, when you decrease your body's inflammatory response, you will also lower your weight and your waist size.

Now do you get the picture and see why it is so important to lose that belly fat?

HIGH CRP LEVELS DON'T ALWAYS MEAN CRISIS

Although elevated CRP levels are associated with an increased risk of cancer, heart disease, diabetes, and hypertension, remember that inflammation is a natural, healthy response to disease, and any infection or injury you suffer will temporarily raise your CRP levels to fight that crisis. Avoid having your CRP levels tested for at least two weeks after you have had an acute infection or suffered an injury to ensure your serum CRP level reflects your actual consistent level and hasn't been spiked due to some recent infection.

Food Allergies and Sensitivities

Given the fat-inflammation connection, it is helpful to know which foods can trigger inflammation and which ones help control it. Some foods trigger inflammation as a matter of course, and we will visit these foods later in the book when we discuss a diet, nutrition, and exercise plan for reducing inflammation. But some foods create inflammation because of our particular food allergies and sensitivities.

Food allergies are a typical inflammatory response often found on the pathway to obesity and diabetes. The most common food allergies are caused by eggs, cow's milk and other dairy products, peanuts, wheat (gluten), soy, tree nuts (such as almonds, cashews, pecans, or walnuts), fish, shellfish, and seeds (sesame and sunflower seeds). An estimated 40 to 50 million Americans have environmental allergies, but only about 4 percent of all adults are allergic to foods or food additives. Among children under the age of four, this increases to 7 percent.[19]

Symptoms of food allergies include hives, eczema, rashes, nausea, vomiting, diarrhea, swollen lips, tingling lips or tongue, stomach cramps, asthma, breathing problems, wheezing, anaphylaxis, and sneezing or a runny, stuffy, or itchy nose. These symptoms usually occur within minutes to a few hours after eating the offending food. Food allergies cause significant inflammation; these substances need to be identified and removed from the diet.

Delayed food sensitivities

Another type of allergy poses significant problems for people trying to manage their weight and blood sugar levels. I have observed that many of my obese patients have delayed food sensitivities. The American Allergy and Immunology Association only allows immunoglobulin E (IgE) reactions to be called "allergy reactions." IgE food allergies produce such symptoms as tingling lips or tongue, swollen lips, or wheezing, generally within minutes to a few hours after eating a food. However, there are three other common yet overlooked allergy pathways. Type II, III, and IV are delayed food reactions, where symptoms may not occur for hours or even days after ingesting the food. Although these delayed allergy reactions are common, patients and physicians often don't recognize them as such because it usually takes awhile for symptoms to occur.

Many cases of obesity and weight gain in which no diet works stem from delayed food sensitivities. Other diseases commonly associated with delayed sensitivities include migraine headaches, psoriasis, irritable bowel syndrome, eczema, arthritis, chronic fatigue syndrome, ADD and ADHD, asthma, fibromyalgia, chronic sinusitis, colitis, Crohn's disease, acid reflux, autism, and rosacea.

Increased intestinal permeability, or leaky gut

Delayed food sensitivities usually start in the intestinal tract when the lining of the GI tract becomes inflamed and hyperpermeable. Some doctors term this increased permeability of the intestinal tract "leaky gut." This simply means that the GI tract has become inflamed. Among the many causes are intestinal infections (food poisoning or bacterial, parasitic, viral, or yeast infections), certain medications (aspirin, anti-inflammatory medications, or antibiotics), or ingesting gut-irritating foods and beverages, such as alcohol or hot spices.

An inflamed gut causes the tight junctions between mucosa cells in the small intestines to open. This allows an increased absorption of partially digested proteins. Under normal circumstances the GI tract only absorbs amino acids (not proteins), glucose, and short-chain fatty acids.

However, with increased intestinal permeability, the body absorbs large food proteins, antigens, and toxins. The body then may produce antibodies against harmless foods that we once enjoyed. Since the body now views these foods as invaders, it forms antibodies to fight them. When IgE antibodies and immune complexes form, they may inflame and damage many different tissues and organs. This eventually leads to the diseases I mentioned above, as well as the inability to lose weight. The most common delayed food sensitivities are dairy, gluten, eggs, peanuts, corn, soy, fish, shellfish, and tree nuts.

Altered GI flora or dysbiosis

Although many bacteria are beneficial, some are potentially pathogenic, meaning they are capable of causing disease. Others are full-fledged pathogens. Pathogenic bacteria often make toxins that can be absorbed back into the bloodstream. Bacterial enzymes can also convert bile into chemicals that promote the development of cancer.

The problem for most people is that because doctors are quick to pull the trigger on prescribing antibiotics, these patients' natural beneficial bacteria levels become imbalanced. When patients use antibiotics too often or for too long, it can create an overabundance of pathogenic bacteria. These upset the natural balance in the large intestine by killing off many beneficial bacteria. This can allow more pathogenic bacteria to grow without restraint.

Under normal circumstances massive amounts of bacteria coexist with significantly smaller colonies of yeast. The excessive number of beneficial bacteria prevents these yeasts from enlarging their territory. However, frequent or prolonged use of antibiotics destroys much of the bacteria and does no harm to the yeast, allowing them to grow unchecked. This can lead to chronic inflammation of the GI tract, food cravings, certain food sensitivities, and weight gain.

Unfortunately, when physicians do not recognize this altered gut ecology, they treat the symptoms while ignoring the root issue. They rarely prescribe beneficial bacteria after taking antibiotics and usually do not limit the patient's sugar intake or consumption of fermented and moldy foods. Yet when patients follow through with these easy steps for just a few months, the problem is usually corrected.

Obviously, treating altered GI ecology is more involved than simply popping a few pills. I incorporated ways to restore the GI tract in my books *Dr. Colbert's "I Can Do This" Diet* and *The Bible Cure for Candida and Yeast Infections*. If this is more problematic for you, I urge you to start replenishing your GI tract with beneficial bacteria through a probiotic (beneficial bacteria). I would also advise you to avoid all sugar and refined foods for at least three months. In my opinion, altered gut ecology is yet another common cause of obesity, setting the stage for diabetes, that often goes unrecognized by traditional medicine.

Action Steps

1. Measure your waistline at your navel. What is that measurement?
2. What is your goal waist measurement?
3. How many times a day do you eat sugars and carbohydrates?
4. Describe how you can reduce that frequency.
5. What foods high in sugar and starch do you need to eliminate from your diet?
6. What foods high in protein and fiber can you add to your diet?
7. What high-glycemic foods can you eliminate?

Chapter 3

DIABETES

When New York filmmaker Morgan Spurlock set out to draw a line between the rise of obesity in America and fast-food giant McDonald's, he never dreamed that his *Super Size Me* documentary would be nominated for an Academy Award, earn more than $20 million worldwide on a $65,000 production budget, and turn the film's title into a watchword for health activists around the globe. In short, he became McDonald's worst nightmare, one accentuated by the release of his ensuing memoir, *Don't Eat This Book.*

Spurlock's unexpected entry into international consciousness originated with a personal experiment, using himself as the guinea pig. For one month he ate nothing but McDonald's food for all three meals, in the process sampling every item on the Golden Arches' menu. Whenever cashiers asked if he wanted his meal supersized, he accepted.

When I first heard of his hypothesis, I found it a bit exaggerated. That is, until I realized that his experiment represented untold millions who get the majority of their daily sustenance from fast food. Spurlock turned himself into a physical representation of these silent masses, consuming an average of 5,000 calories a day. As a result, he gained almost 25 pounds, increased his body mass index by 13 percent, raised his cholesterol to 230, and accumulated fat in his liver. He turned his experiment into a statement heard around the world.[1]

Years later I sometimes wonder if many Americans were paying attention. After reports in recent years of a stabilization in obesity rates, a report released by the Centers for Disease Control and Prevention in the summer of 2011 showed they had inched up 1.1 percent between 2007 and 2009, leaving them at staggering levels of 33.8 percent.[2] The proportion of obese American adults is at astounding levels, more than one-third, or 34.9 percent.[3] Obesity currently kills an estimated four hundred thousand Americans a year and is the second-leading cause of preventable deaths in this nation.[4] The number one avoidable killer? Cigarette smoking (and a recent report shows it dropped 40 percent between 1965 and 2007).[5] That means losing weight ranks up there with quitting smoking as the most crucial lifestyle change you could ever make. Because of the lowered smoking trend, I predict that obesity will soon pass smoking as the number one avoidable killer of Americans.

Unfortunately, many doctors, nutritionists, and dietitians seem to either miss this fact or conveniently ignore it. They love to offer topical "Band-Aids" that alleviate patients' symptoms yet fail to tackle the root issues or consider the long-term ramifications of neglecting their patients' weight. A CDC report in 2007 found that about a third of obese adults had never been told by a doctor or health-care provider that they were obese.[6] Not only is this unbelievable, but obesity is also a key link to another serious, life-threatening issue: diabetes.

Diabetes kills more people than AIDS and breast cancer combined. It reportedly ranks as the seventh leading cause of death by disease among adults in America.[7] The sad reality is that it may rank much higher because research shows that diabetes is underreported, only being listed on 10 to 15 percent of death certificates as an underlying cause of death.[8]

NATIONAL SUGAR HIGH

In the early 1980s roughly one in seven Americans was obese and almost 6 million were diabetic. By the early 2000s, when national sugar consumption hit its peak, one in three Americans was obese and 14 million were diabetic.[9]

In 2011, the World Health Organization reported that 347 million people had diabetes. They went on to estimate that by 2030 diabetes will be the seventh leading cause of death worldwide.[10] And within the United States type 2 diabetes is increasing at an alarming rate. Not only do approximately one in every ten Americans age twenty and older have diabetes,[11] but also the rate of children being diagnosed with type 2 diabetes is growing at a frightening rate.

Such alarming information speaks for itself. Indeed, it is screaming while far too many practitioners turn the other way. With our nation facing the biggest health-care crisis in its history, each of us must realize that the answer won't come from doctors, clinics, or the US government. Instead, each person must take responsibility for his or her health. And because obesity and overweight conditions are at the root of diabetes, it makes sense to learn about this disease, its causes and early warning signs, its connection to inflammation, and how to go about reversing its onset.

The Often-Silent Killer

Nearly 26 million American adults suffer from this disease called diabetes—and a fourth of them don't even know they have it![12] Researchers at the Centers for Disease Control and Prevention recently made the stunning revelation that during the 2005–2008 time period, 35 percent of US adults age twenty or older had prediabetes, including 50 percent of those over sixty-five. Applying those percentages to the entire population yields an estimated 79 million Americans with prediabetes. Add diabetics and prediabetics together, and approximately one-third of our population, or 103 million, have prediabetes or diabetes.

In addition, some 215,000 people under age twenty have type 1 or type 2 diabetes, the latter formerly considered an adult-onset problem. The CDC had already projected that without changes in diet and exercise, one in three children born in the United States in the year 2000 are likely to develop type 2 diabetes at some point during their lives.[13]

Why are we seeing such dramatic increases? It can be traced directly to what we discussed in the last chapter: the nation's obesity epidemic. To offer the primary statistics again, two-thirds of American adults are overweight or obese, and 30 percent of children age eleven or younger are overweight.[14] Simply put, the lifestyle changes prevalent in our culture give rise to obesity and the onset of diabetes. Galatians 6:7–8 says, "Be not deceived. God is not mocked. For whatever a man sows, that will he also reap. For the one who sows to his own flesh will from the flesh reap corruption, but the one who sows to the Spirit will from the Spirit reap eternal life." Most Americans are unknowingly sowing seeds for a harvest of obesity, diabetes, and a host of other diseases by their choices of food and lifestyle habits.

The additionally unfortunate truth, however, is that many physicians are looking for the next new-and-improved medication to cure all ills. I suggest that is not a solution. We need to get to the root of the problem, which is our diet, lifestyle, and waistline—all of which we will discuss in detail in the latter half of this book. Without addressing the reality of these factors, the alarming toll from diabetes will only get worse.

Globesity Is the Culprit

According to author Michael Pollan, diabetes subtracts roughly twelve years from one's life, while someone living with the condition incurs annual medical costs of $13,000, compared to $2,500 for a person without diabetes. And although an estimated 80 percent of cases of type 2 diabetes are preventable with proper diet and exercise, he says the smart money is on the creation of a vast new industry: "Apparently it is easier, or at least a lot more profitable, to change a disease of civilization into a lifestyle than it is to change the way that civilization eats."[15]

Tragically, millions of others outside the United States struggle with the same issues. The World Health Organization calls obesity a worldwide epidemic. Obesity and its expanding list of health consequences—led by diabetes—is overtaking infection and malnutrition as the main cause of death and disability in many third-world nations. This "globesity," as Morgan Spurlock aptly points out in his documentary, has a major cause: the spread of fast food.

In his award-winning book *Fast Food Nation* author Eric Schlosser chronicles how Americans spent about $6 billion on fast food in 1970 but by the turn of the century shelled out more than $110 billion. Because corporate America is a global trend-setter, other countries have followed suit. Between 1984 and 1993 the number of fast-food restaurants in Great Britain doubled. So did adults' obesity rate. Fast-forward fifteen years, and the British were eating more fast food than any other nation in Western Europe.

MEN, WAIST SIZE, AND TYPE 2 DIABETES

The larger your waist, the greater your chances of having type 2 diabetes. For men, waist size is an even better predictor of diabetes than BMI. A thirteen-year study of more than twenty-seven thousand men discovered that:

- A waist size of 34 to 36 inches doubled diabetes risk.
- A waist size of 36 to 38 nearly tripled the risk.
- A waist size of 38 to 40 was associated with five times the risk.
- A waist size of 40 to 62 was associated with twelve times the risk.[16]

Meanwhile the proportion of overweight teens in China has roughly tripled in the past decade. In Japan the obesity rate among children doubled during the 1980s, which correlated with a 200 percent increase in fast-food sales. This generation of Japanese has gone on to become the first in that traditionally slender Asian nation's history—thanks to its past proclivity for vegetables, rice, and fish—to be known for its bulging waistlines. By the year 2000 approximately one-third of all Japanese men in their thirties were overweight.[17] By adopting our fast-food habits, the entire world is beginning to look more like Americans. I fear that its diabetes rates will soon follow.

A Child Shall Lead Them

How has an entire generation of hefty eaters changed the face of the world? By starting young. Once again this unflattering trend originated in America. As I mentioned above, according to a 2011 CDC report, nearly 26 million Americans have diabetes, or 8.3 percent of the US population. And again, in an earlier report, the CDC projected that one out of three children who were born in the United States in the year 2000 will develop type 2 diabetes at some point in their life.[18]

As a result of childhood obesity, the numbers of children with type 2 diabetes are rapidly rising across the country. And because of the connection of obesity to hypertension, high cholesterol, and heart disease, experts are predicting a dramatic rise in heart disease as our children become adults. The CDC reports that overweight teens stand a 70 percent chance of becoming overweight adults, which increases to 80 percent if at least one parent is obese or overweight. Because of that, heart disease and type 2 diabetes are expected to begin at a much earlier age among those who fail to beat the odds.[19] Today's generation of children is not expected to live as long as their parents, and they will be more likely to suffer from disease and illness at an earlier age.

TRENDS IN CHILDHOOD OBESITY

Research shows that childhood obesity more than doubled in children and quadrupled in adolescents over the past thirty years. Obesity among children ages six to eleven jumped from 7 percent in 1980 to almost 18 percent in 2012. The rate rose even faster for those twelve to nineteen, increasing from 5 percent to 21 percent. Seventy percent of obese youth have at least one risk for cardiovascular disease. They are also likely to become obese adults, increasing their risk of associated health problems—diabetes among them.[20]

So if you don't want to lose weight and reverse the onset of diabetes for yourself, at least do it for your children. Children follow by example by mirroring their parents' behavior. Don't tell them to live healthy if you aren't doing it yourself. I'm sure most of you are good parents and love your children. Yet you have to ask yourself: "Do I love them enough to teach them what foods to eat and what foods to avoid? Do I love them enough to keep junk food out of the house while making healthy food available? Do I love them enough to engage in physical activity and lead by example?"

If you answered yes to those questions, it is important that you take action for your children's sake—and your own. This is not a "crash diet, quick fix" method but permanent lifestyle changes. You hold the key to truly changing your life and reversing the onset of diabetes, whether yours or the early signs appearing in your children. However, to be frank, this will not be an easy fight when it involves your children. They are growing up in a culture saturated with junk food that is void of nutrition and high in toxic fats, sugar, highly processed carbohydrates, and food additives and that is not only widely available but also heavily advertised.

To add to the challenge, they are surrounded by peers who consider consuming this junk natural and a normal part of childhood. For example, in 1978 the typical teen male in the United States drank 7 ounces of soda a day; today he drinks approximately three times that much. Meanwhile he gets about a quarter of his daily servings of vegetables from french fries and potato chips.[21]

YOUNG AND SWEET

Sugary-sweet cereals were introduced in the early 1950s, when companies first targeted children in their advertisements. Among the first cereals to debut was Kellogg's aptly named Sugar Smacks, which contained an astounding 56 percent sugar.[22] The company later renamed the product Honey Smacks, but don't let that name fool you; sugar is still the number one ingredient on its label.

If you plan to take a stand against this garbage-in, garbage-out culture, expect opposition on every front. During the course of a year the typical American child will watch more than thirty thousand TV commercials, many of them pitching fast food or junk food as delicious "must-eats." For years fast-food franchises have enticed children into their restaurants with kids' meal toys, promotional giveaways, and elaborate playgrounds. This has worked perfectly for McDonald's: about 90 percent of American children between the ages of three and nine set foot in one each month.[23] When they can't visit the Golden Arches or another favored outlet, it comes to them. Fast-food products—most brought in by franchisees—are sold in about 30 percent of public high school cafeterias and many elementary cafeterias.[24]

Because they spend billions of dollars on research and marketing, these fast-food establishments know exactly what they are doing and how to push your child's hot button. They understand the powerful impact certain foods can have on people at an early age. Have you ever thought about when you first started liking certain foods? Most people formed these preferences during the first few years of their lives. This is why comfort foods often do more than just fill the stomach. They evoke such memories as playgrounds, toys, backyard birthday bashes, Fourth of July parties, state fairs, and childhood friends. The aroma of onion rings, doughnuts, or grilled burgers can instantly trigger these memories. As adults, such smells often draw us without us recognizing their lure. Advertisers have keyed into this and learned to use the sight of food to stimulate fond childhood memories.

In the Genes or in the Water?

Every obese person has a story behind his or her excessive weight gain. Growing up, I often heard people say things such as "she was born fat" or "he takes after his daddy."

There's some truth in both comments. When it comes to obesity, genetics count. In 1986 the *New England Journal of Medicine* published a Danish study that observed 540 people adopted during infancy. The research found that adopted individuals had a much greater tendency to end up in the weight class of their biological parents rather than their adoptive parents.[25] Separate studies of twins raised apart also show that genetics has a strong influence on weight gain and becoming overweight.[26] Such studies reveal there is a significant genetic predisposition to gaining weight.

However, they still don't fully explain the epidemic of obesity seen in the United States the past thirty years. Although an individual may have a genetic predisposition to become obese, environment also plays a major role. I like the way author, speaker, and noted women's physician Pamela Peeke puts it: "Genetics may load the gun, but environment pulls the trigger."[27] Many patients I see come into my office thinking that since they have inherited their "fat genes," there is nothing they can do to lose weight or reverse the diseases headed their way, type 2 diabetes among them. Yet after a little investigation I usually find that they have inherited their parents' propensity for bad food choices, large portion sizes, and poor eating habits.

FAST FACT

More than 90 percent of people who are newly diagnosed with type 2 diabetes are overweight or obese.[28]

If you have been overweight since childhood, you probably have an increased number of fat cells. This means you will have a tendency to gain weight if you choose the wrong types of foods and large portions and fail to exercise. It also means you will have a greater chance of incurring type 2 diabetes. However, you should also realize that most people can override a genetic predisposition for diabetes by making correct dietary and lifestyle choices. A parent's diabetes does not automatically condemn a child to the same disease, no matter how many people remark, "The apple doesn't fall far from the tree."

Unfortunately, many of us forget that to make these healthy choices, we need to place ourselves in a healthy environment. That is becoming more difficult than ever as families yield to hectic routines that feature grabbing breakfast on the way out the door, fast-food lunches, dining out for dinner, and sometimes skipping meals. Years of such habits are catching up to us. Starting at age twenty-five, the average American adult gains 1 to 3 pounds a year. That means a twenty-five-year-old, 120-pound female can expect to weigh anywhere between 150 and 210 pounds by the time she is fifty-five.

Is there any wonder we have an epidemic of type 2 diabetes in our nation? We have to put the brakes on this obesity epidemic—and a lifestyle approach to eating is the answer!

THE SIMPLE FACT

People suffering from diabetes have high sugar levels in their blood.

Eat With the Head, Not the Heart

The fact that obesity and a predisposition to diabetes can stem from heredity, environment, and culture can feel discouraging, even overwhelming. How can one hope to overcome such powerful forces and reverse diabetes in the process?

As tough as it may seem, there is cause for hope. It may sound impossible, but with education, practice, and discipline your cultural tastes and dietary practices can gradually change. You can learn to choose similar foods that have not been highly processed and lower-fat alternatives. It is possible to discover—or rediscover—portion control and healthy cooking methods. What about fried chicken, mashed potatoes and gravy, and chocolate cake? You can learn to enjoy the same foods but with just a fraction of the fat, sugar, and calories. The real pleasure in most foods is in the first few bites.

If you remember nothing else from this book, remember this truth: you can break old, culturally based eating patterns. You do not have to follow a parent's poor food choices, and you can overcome your family's dietary cultural patterns. (I certainly did!) In the process you will discover the true joy of eating.

The Proof Is in the Urine

The iPad and similar twenty-first-century notebooks are so prevalent today that some companies and organizations require that employees carry them to seminars and conferences. Watch televised election returns from the latest presidential or congressional races, and you will see the anchors and field reporters checking electronic updates, whether on an electronic notebook or smartphone. Small wonder that the assumption is that everyone in the modern era checks their apps and other devices to stay abreast of up-to-the-minute developments, even as young adults show signs that they are stressed out by the flood of gizmos they are expected to master. In the fall of 2010 an annual survey of college freshmen by UCLA showed their emotional health had fallen to its lowest levels in twenty-five years.[29]

It's ironic, then, that thousands of years ago the laid-back Romans and Greeks—who wrote on wax-coated tablets with a stylus made of metal, bone, or ivory—possessed an understanding of diabetes even though they had no blood tests for them. Though it may sound gross to modern sensibilities, the Romans and Greeks could detect diabetes by simply tasting a person's urine. Yech! Though I wonder who mastered this breakthrough (and especially how they did so), they discovered that some people's urine had a sweet taste, or *mellitus*—the Latin word for *sweet*. In addition, the Greeks realized that when patients with sweet urine drank any fluids, they generally excreted these fluids in their urine almost as rapidly as they went in the mouth, similar to a siphon. In fact, the Greek word for *siphon* is *diabetes*. So now you know how we got the name *diabetes mellitus*. It all started by tasting the urine. I, for one, am glad that doctors abandoned this practice and that we can check a patient's blood sugar today!

I have good news for you too: not only is this disease thousands of years old, but also so is God's power to heal. Just as God healed the sick thousands of years ago in the days of the Bible, He still heals today. He has also provided a wealth of proven biblical principles and invaluable medical knowledge about the human body. You can control the symptoms and potentially damaging effects of diabetes while you seek Him for total healing. You are destined to be more than a victim. You are destined to be a victor in this battle!

Your first order of battle in attacking the symptoms of diabetes, or prediabetes, is to know your enemy. After measuring its strengths, plan for ways you can defeat it. The enemy known as diabetes comes in many forms.

The Choice Disease

Diabetes is actually a group of diseases including type 1 diabetes, type 2 diabetes, prediabetes, and gestational diabetes. Each type is characterized by high levels of blood sugar that is the result of either defective insulin production, defects in the action of insulin, or both.

The onset of type 1 diabetes is beyond anyone's control. However, I often say that prediabetes and type 2 diabetes are "choice" diseases. In other words, you catch a cold or the flu, but because of wrong choices, you develop obesity, prediabetes, and type 2 diabetes.

Type 1 diabetes

In the past, type 1 diabetes was called insulin-dependent diabetes, juvenile-onset diabetes, or childhood-onset diabetes. Although it can strike at any age, this form usually occurs in children or young adults. In adults it is quite rare, with only approximately 5 percent of all cases of diabetes proving to be type 1 diabetes.[30]

While we do not have all the pieces of the puzzle for this type of diabetes, risk factors may be genetic or environmental. Some researchers believe that the environmental trigger is probably a virus. Others believe the trigger may be ingesting protein from cow's milk, especially during infancy. In my book *Eat This and Live! for Kids*, Dr. Joseph Cannizzaro and I recommend increasing your child's intake of vitamin D, reducing intake of cow's milk, limiting or avoiding gluten, and avoiding all nitrates and nitrites to prevent type 1 diabetes.

What we do know about type 1 diabetes is that it is caused by the body's immune system attacking itself and eventually destroying the beta cells in the pancreas. The beta cells are the only cells in the body that make insulin, which is the hormone that regulates blood sugar. Patients with type 1 diabetes require insulin either by injection or by an insulin pump in order to survive.

Over the years my patients with type 1 diabetes who have maintained the best blood sugar control have been those using an insulin pump. Newer insulin pumps have remote controls, making it much easier to control your blood sugar. In treating patients, I have discovered that dietary and lifestyle changes and nutritional supplements will usually lower insulin requirements in type 1 diabetics, but they will still require insulin. Once you begin such a program, it is necessary to monitor your blood sugar daily, adjust your insulin accordingly, and follow up with your physician on a regular basis.

The hemoglobin A1C test is the best way to monitor your blood sugar over the long run. Hemoglobin is a protein that carries oxygen in the blood. It is present inside the red blood cells that live only for about 90 to 120 days. The hemoglobin A1C measures how much glucose has entered the red blood cells and become stuck to the hemoglobin, similar to a fly stuck to flypaper.[31] If someone has a high blood sugar level throughout the day, more sugar will stick to the hemoglobin. If blood sugar is typically only slightly elevated during the day, less sugar will stick to the hemoglobin, and the hemoglobin A1C will be lower.

Most diabetes specialists recommend that diabetic patients strive to lower their hemoglobin A1C to 6.5 percent or less to prevent most of the complications of diabetes. They also recommend that patients take this blood test every three to four months. I personally try to get my diabetic patients' hemoglobin A1C to around 6 percent or less because at this level, I find that they rarely ever develop severe complications.

If you are battling type 1 diabetes, continue to follow your doctor's advice, continue to take your insulin, and consult your doctor before making any lifestyle or nutritional changes. In addition, determine to believe God—who created your pancreas—for a miraculous touch of healing power. The Word of God says, "For with God nothing will be impossible" (Luke 1:37).

Remember that faith is not a feeling or an emotion; it is a choice. Specifically ask the Lord to heal your pancreas and restore its ability to manufacture insulin. Jesus said in Mark 9:23, "All things are possible to him who believes," and in Mark 10:27, "For with God all things are possible."

CAUSE AND EFFECT

According to the American Diabetes Association, diabetes is now:

- The leading cause of kidney failure, accounting for 44 percent of cases in 2008
- Responsible for a heart disease death rate two to four times higher among diabetics than adults without diabetes
- The leading cause of new blindness cases among people ages twenty to seventy-four
- Responsible for more than 60 percent of non-traumatic, lower-limb amputations
- Responsible for mild to severe forms of nervous system damage in 60–70 percent of all diabetics[32]

Prediabetes

A person does not just wake up one day with type 2 diabetes. Developing it is a slow, insidious process that usually takes years to a decade to develop. It always starts with prediabetes.

Prediabetes (formerly called *borderline* or *subclinical diabetes*) is a condition in which a person's blood glucose or hemoglobin A1C levels are higher than normal but not high enough to be diagnosed as diabetes. People with prediabetes have a greater risk of developing type 2 diabetes, heart disease, and stroke. From 2005 to 2008, based on fasting glucose or hemoglobin A1C levels, 35 percent of US adults had prediabetes. Applying this percentage to the entire US population in 2010 puts the estimate at 79 million adults with prediabetes.[33]

Diabetes is defined as a fasting blood sugar level greater than or equal to 126 mg/dL or a casual blood sugar level (usually after eating) greater than or equal to 200 mg/dL. High blood sugar levels are usually accompanied by symptoms of diabetes, including frequent urination, excessive thirst, and changes in vision.[34]

People with prediabetes typically have impaired glucose tolerance, impaired fasting glucose, or both. Often they do not know they have prediabetes. And it typically takes years—sometimes even more than a decade—to progress from prediabetes into full-blown type 2 diabetes.

Type 2 diabetes

Type 2 diabetes was previously called *non-insulin-dependent diabetes* or *adult-onset diabetes.* That's because, historically, most people contracted the disease in their adult years. Sadly our nation's taste for high-sugar, high-fat diets seems to have removed age barriers. In recent years the medical community has reported that this form of diabetes accounts for a growing number of juvenile cases. In adults, 90 to 95 percent of all diabetes cases are type 2 diabetes.[35] And, according to the CDC, 1.9 million new cases of diabetes in people twenty and older were diagnosed in 2010.[36]

Type 2 diabetes is more of a genetic disease than type 1. However, although genetic makeup may have "loaded the gun," environmental factors like belly fat, poor diet, and lifestyle will, again, "pull the trigger." Stop playing the blame game. Face your need to change. If you're in danger of developing diabetes or have crossed the line, recognize that losing belly fat, controlling your diet, and exercising regularly means you will probably never develop diabetes or can usually reverse it. Take heart from the major diabetes prevention study that revealed that lifestyle changes reduced developing diabetes by more than 70 percent of high-risk people who were over sixty years old.[37]

By the time people develop type 2 diabetes, they typically experience such bothersome symptoms as increased thirst, increased urination, frequent nighttime urination, blurred vision, or fatigue. Type 2 diabetes is typically associated with obesity (especially truncal, which refers to fat deposits in the torso and abdomen), increasing age, a family history of diabetes, physical inactivity, or a history of gestational diabetes. Race or ethnic heritage also plays a role in risk factors. American Indians, Hispanic Americans, African Americans, and some Asian Americans and Pacific Islanders have a higher chance of developing type 2 diabetes and its complications.

Gestational diabetes

Although acquired during pregnancy, gestational diabetes only occurs in about 2 percent of pregnancies. This form of diabetes is due to the growing fetus and placenta secreting hormones that decrease the body's sensitivity to insulin, which can lead to diabetes.

If a woman develops gestational diabetes, it usually goes away after giving birth. Only 5 to 10 percent of women with gestational diabetes are found to have type 2 diabetes after giving birth. However, this form of diabetes increases a woman's risk of developing type 2 diabetes later in life. Studies show that women who have had gestational diabetes have a 35 to 60 percent chance of developing type 2 diabetes within ten to twenty years after pregnancy.[38] Gestational diabetes occurs more frequently among African Americans, American Indians, and Hispanic Americans.

A caution here: don't take your presence in one of these groups as evidence that you are bound for trouble. Still, it can be a signal that you need to pay closer attention to diet, exercise, and losing belly fat. Such advice can be repeated for everyone in our "couch potato" nation.

Inflammation and Diabetes

For years, when explaining diabetes to patients, I have said that insulin is like a key that unlocks the door to your cells. Type 2 diabetes is similar to having rusty locks on those cells. Every cell in your body needs sugar. The hormone insulin removes sugar from the bloodstream and binds to insulin receptors on the surface of the cells, similar to a key unlocking a lock and opening the door. The insulin opens the door to the cells (figuratively speaking) and allows sugar to enter.

The majority of people who develop type 2 diabetes still produce insulin; however, the cells in their bodies do not use the insulin properly. In type 2 diabetics the cells resist insulin's normal function. This condition is known as *insulin resistance.* It is as though the key goes in to unlock the lock, but just like a rusty lock, the insulin does not work as well. If you have ever tried to open an old, rust-encrusted lock, you will understand this analogy. Over time this insulin resistance leads to prediabetes and type 2 diabetes.

Now, remember what I said in the last chapter about the connection between fat and inflammation, how these two factors get caught in a vicious trap? Weight gain leads to inflammation, which leads to further weight gain, which leads to further inflammation.

Inflammation has been found to be one of the key factors leading to insulin resistance in the body's cells. When the key can't open the lock, chronic inflammation is one reason why. Due to that inflammation the lock can't open, which means insulin can't get through the door of the cells to allow sugar in.

When the difficulty with lock and key happens, insulin levels then begin to rise as your body needs more and more insulin to allow sugar to enter the cells. This is similar to jiggling a key over and over until it springs the rusty lock. That means an excessive amount of insulin is needed to keep blood sugar levels in the normal range. Eventually, as cells become more and more insulin resistant, higher insulin levels are unable to lower the blood sugar. The blood sugar rises higher and higher, meaning the individual develops prediabetes and eventually type 2 diabetes.

Insulin resistance is the main cause of type 2 diabetes. Though usually a manageable problem, it is complicated by the fact that truncal obesity is one of the most important factors leading to insulin resistance. Obese people with type 2 diabetes must decrease their belly fat by choosing low-glycemic foods. This means that type 2 diabetics require a diet that:

- Is low in refined processed starches, such as white rice, white bread, potatoes, and pasta
- Contains very little sugar

Notice the Warning Signs

"Listen to your body" is an adage that many doctors pass along to their patients. Although this is not a foolproof method—especially considering my previous observation that someone with prediabetes won't necessarily notice any symptoms—you should pay attention to any warning signs that physical trouble is brewing. There are countless numbers of people lying in the cemetery who passed off chest pains or other obvious signs of heart trouble as indigestion. Or they didn't want to bother anyone or take the time to go to the doctor. Ignore your body, and you could soon be pushing up daisies.

As with most diseases, early detection of diabetes is crucial. Silent enemies sometimes inflict the most damage. Fortunately, for some people, diabetes has telltale symptoms, which are listed below (note that these aren't restricted to age or gender). Don't panic just because you have noticed one of these symptoms. Some may occur periodically simply because you drank too much liquid one night, ate some spicy food, or stayed up too late. However, if you experience one or more of these symptoms on a regular basis, make an appointment with your physician to get screened for diabetes and prediabetes. Then you can apply the truths in this book and in God's Word to the situation. Above all, don't give in to fear or apathy.

Type 1 diabetes

- Frequent urination
- Unusual thirst
- Extreme hunger
- Unusual weight loss
- Extreme fatigue and irritability[39]

Type 2 diabetes*

- Any of the type 1 symptoms
- Frequent infections
- Blurred vision
- Cuts/bruises that are slow to heal
- Tingling/numbness in the hands/feet
- Recurring skin, gum, or bladder infections[40]

Treatable and Beatable

As with most diseases, serious health complications occur when someone with diabetes fails to do anything about this very treatable—and beatable—disease. The more serious complications of diabetes include diabetic retinopathy (the leading cause of blindness in the United States), diabetic neuropathy (a degeneration of peripheral nerves that leads to tingling, numbness, pain, and weakness usually in extremities such as the legs and feet), kidney disease, and atherosclerosis or arteriosclerosis. Approximately 20–25 percent will develop either impaired kidney function or kidney failure on average of eleven years after diagnosis.[41]

* Sometimes people with type 2 diabetes have no symptoms.

DIABETES AND THE HEART

Arteriosclerosis is hardening of the arteries. Atherosclerosis is when arteriosclerosis occurs due to fatty deposits on the inner lining of the arterial walls. Approximately 44 percent of diabetics will develop atherosclerosis of the carotid arteries and in peripheral arteries. Diabetics are approximately two to five times at greater risk of a heart attack or coronary artery disease compared to nondiabetics.[42]

Proponents of eating meat often point to Genesis 9:3, where God gave mankind the freedom to consume meat. What these advocates fail to appreciate is that the average American's excessive consumption of meat, as well as carbohydrates, sugar, and fat, can cause numerous health problems. Diabetics—particularly those who fail to control their insulin and blood sugar levels through proper diet, exercise, and lifestyle choices—are much more prone to heart disease, heart attacks, kidney disease (a primary cause of death in diabetics), foot ulcers (usually due to poor blood supply), and peripheral nerve disease in the feet.

In what can only be called a burst of wishful thinking, most people with diabetes think they will never develop long-term complications. They rationalize that they will surely have early signs and symptoms before they develop these terrible complications. Or they assume they will be able to take medications that will reverse the impact of the disease.

I tell my patients that diabetes is similar to a house infested with termites. When termites have been eating away at a home for long enough, one day when the homeowner tries to hang a picture on a wall, a gaping hole may suddenly appear. Or a door suddenly sticks, and when the homeowner pushes on the door, the frame caves in. Now, this does not happen immediately. Termite-inflicted damage takes months or even years to surface, but the impact is unmistakable.

Poorly controlled diabetes is a silent killer that works in a way similar to termites. After many years, sometimes decades, terrible health conditions suddenly begin to surface thanks to long-term diabetes. While medications can slow the process or control some of the symptoms, they usually do not get to the root of the problem. This makes Michael Pollan's observation about America's "solution" of turning a disease into a lifestyle an apt commentary on the folly of our nation's approach to our health crisis. Long-term elevation of blood sugar eventually damages and destroys the beta cells of the pancreas, which are the insulin-producing cells. Oxidative stress and chronic inflammation will also eventually damage and destroy the insulin-producing cells. The longer these processes go on (high blood sugar, chronic inflammation, and oxidative stress), the more beta cells will die. Eventually, when the number of beta cells is half of their original number, type 2 diabetes is then typically irreversible. That is why it is so important to identify prediabetes and type 2 diabetes and lower the blood sugar as well as the inflammation before permanent damage is done.

The Danger of Useless Trash

The main reason diabetics develop complications such as heart attacks, peripheral vascular disease, kidney disease, neuropathy, eye disease, and erectile dysfunction is because of the accumulation of advanced glycation end-products (AGEs). The higher the blood sugar and the longer the time the blood sugar is elevated, the more AGEs will accumulate. The sugar (glucose) molecule reacts with any free amino groups of proteins, lipids, and nucleic acids and forms AGEs. AGEs form crosslinks between proteins, which alter their structure and function.

AGEs are the root cause of almost all complications of diabetes, including retinopathy, neuropathy, nephropathy (kidney disease), and atherosclerosis. AGEs in tissues increase the rate of free radical production fifty times the rate of unglycated proteins. AGEs attach to LDL cholesterol, increasing oxidation of the cholesterol and leading to plaque in the arteries or atherosclerosis. They also accumulate in the kidneys, nerves, eyes (lens and blood vessels), brain (accelerating brain cell death), skin (forming wrinkles and sagging skin), blood vessels and nerves of the penis (accelerating erectile dysfunction), as well as in all muscles, organs, and tissues throughout the body.

AGEs are simply useless cellular trash or debris that eventually damages and destroys tissues and organs as they accumulate. They have no beneficial function at all and cannot be utilized for energy. Once they form, they are irreversible and cannot be repaired, detoxified, or removed from the body.

This is why long-term elevation of blood sugar is so dangerous. You are accelerating the aging process and accumulating cellular debris that will eventually impair and destroy many different tissues in the body as they accumulate. The higher the blood sugar, the more AGEs will accumulate, which literally invites a host of deadly diseases into your body and accelerates the aging process.

I wish people could comprehend that in a prediabetic or diabetic patient, that slice of cake, piece of pie, fudge, brownie, candy bar, or soda is raising the blood sugar and creating irreversible AGEs. The AGEs in turn are wrinkling your skin, causing erectile dysfunction in men, and setting you up for cardiovascular disease, kidney disease that eventually may require dialysis, and peripheral neuropathy, in which you may develop numbness and tingling or burning pains in your feet and extremities. Are you getting the picture?

Marketers have glamorized sugary items, and oh, how attractive and enticing are the birthday cakes and pastries when you enter the bakery section of any grocery store as you inhale that wonderful aroma of freshly baked pastries. But then go to a dialysis unit where patients typically have to be dialyzed three times a week for three hours a treatment, and you will find the majority of those patients are diabetic. Only you can start to make the correct choices.

DR. COLBERT APPROVED—HEMOGLOBIN TEST

There is a simple blood test to gauge your rate of AGE formation, and it's called the hemoglobin A1C test or HbA1C. This is a very common test used to monitor a diabetic's blood sugar over a few months, but it can also monitor glycation in a prediabetic patient or even healthy patients without prediabetes or diabetes. I am amazed at how many of my (so-called) healthy weight patients have an elevated HbA1C and don't even realize it. They are eating desserts and drinking sodas, and because they are not overweight or obese, they think they are healthy. However, they are forming AGEs, which are accumulating and accelerating the aging process.

Most nondiabetic Americans have an HbA1C of 5.0 percent to 6.4 percent. If the HbA1C is greater than 6.5, the patient has diabetes. Approximately 70 percent of American adults have an HbA1C between 5.0 percent and 6.9 percent.[43]

What most people do not realize is that the HbA1C does not have to be 6.5 or higher to cause health problems. Every 1 percent increase in HbA1C, even when the HbA1C was in the normal range, was associated with an increased risk of heart attacks, cancer, and increased mortality.

I believe the optimum HbA1C is 6 percent or less, since this is the normal rate of glycation. Quite a few diabetics have an HbA1C of 10, which is almost twice the normal rate of glycation. The higher the HbA1C, simply speaking, the faster you are aging.

Don't Sign for It

Is this helping you get the picture? Habitual consumption of soft drinks, candy bars, pie or cake, or large helpings of white rice, potatoes, and white bread will increase inflammation in your body and help you sign on the dotted line for prediabetes and diabetes.

Over the years I have seen patients stressed out over signing a contract without reading the small print. A few years ago a patient came in burning with anger because after moving out of his apartment, he discovered that he owed the owners an extra $1,000. He said that he never had to pay after leaving other apartment complexes. The manager replied, "Read your contract." When he did, my patient saw the extra-fine print that stipulated when an occupant left his apartment, he would have to pay $1,000.

In the same way millions of Americans are unknowingly signing up for diabetes, accompanied by all of the complications associated with this disease. Wake up. Take action while there is still time to reverse the curse of prediabetes and diabetes.

Action Steps

1. Which of these diabetes symptoms do you have?
    - Frequent urination
    - Unusual thirst
    - Extreme hunger
    - Unusual weight loss
    - Extreme fatigue and irritability
    - Frequent infections
    - Blurred vision
    - Cuts/bruises that are slow to heal
    - Tingling/numbness in the hands/feet
    - Recurring skin, gum, or bladder infections
2. What did you eat today?
    - Breakfast
    - Morning snack(s)
    - Lunch
    - Afternoon snack(s)
    - Dinner
    - Evening snack(s)
3. Now go through your food list above, noting the living, healthy foods and the dead, unhealthy foods.
4. Make a plan for your eating schedule tomorrow:
    - Breakfast
    - Morning snack(s)
    - Lunch
    - Afternoon snack(s)
    - Dinner
    - Evening snack(s)

Chapter 4

ARTHRITIS

Arthritis pain is not new. Did you know that arthritis is one of the earliest documented afflictions in history? Scientists have discovered evidence of arthritis in the bones of mummies from the pyramids of ancient Egypt.

But this ancient disease has a remedy older than history—the Ancient of Days, who is God our healer. For millennia people have suffered unnecessarily. God has not only provided many natural ways for you to be relieved of arthritic pain caused by inflammation, but He has also provided supernatural healing for your body through trusting His Word and drawing near to Him. Listen to His promise:

> If you diligently heed the voice of the Lord your God and do what is right in His sight, give ear to His commandments and keep all His statutes, I will put none of the diseases on you which I have brought on the Egyptians. For I am the Lord who heals you.
>
> —Exodus 15:26

God understands your pain and suffering. In fact, the Bible talks specifically about arthritis pain. The biblical songwriter may be echoing your feelings exactly when he wrote, "I am poured out like water, and all my bones are out of joint; my heart is like wax; it has melted within Me.... I can count all My bones" (Ps. 22:14, 17). Not only does God understand your pain, but He has also provided natural, medical, and spiritual ways for you to overcome your arthritis pain and be healed. God your healer desires for you to be physically healthy so that you can enjoy life to its fullest and serve Him. Let's learn how reversing inflammation is a part of that process and what you can do to soothe your aching and burning joints.

Let's begin by determining what kind of arthritis pain you have.

What's Your Joint Issue?

Are you suffering with rheumatoid arthritis—called an autoimmune disease because your symptoms are caused by your body's immune system attacking itself? Or have you been diagnosed with osteoarthritis—caused by the degeneration of your joints and the loss of cartilage? While there are many different forms of arthritis, these are its two main forms.

Osteoarthritis

Osteoarthritis is by far the most common form of arthritis. It is also termed *degenerative joint disease* and is most often characterized by joint pain. The joint pain is due to a gradual loss of cartilage and degeneration of the joint. An estimated 27 million Americans suffer from it.[1] Osteoarthritis primarily affects the larger weight-bearing joints. Approximately a third of Americans over the age of sixty-five suffer from this form of arthritis.[2] And there are two main forms of it: primary and secondary.

Primary osteoarthritis usually begins after the age of forty-five, affecting the fingers, neck, lower back, knees, and hips. While the cause is unknown, we do know that obese individuals tend to develop it more commonly. As you gain weight, the pressure on the weight-bearing joints such as the hips and knees increases dramatically. When an obese patient runs or jumps, the pressure on the joints can be as much as ten times a person's body weight. In other words, if a 250-pound man jumped down off of a ladder, the pressure on his hips and knees could be as much as a ton! Is there any wonder why patients who are obese are becoming crippled with osteoarthritis?

Secondary osteoarthritis is simply due to trauma. I commonly see ex-football players in my practice who are crippled with osteoarthritis, especially in the fingers and the knees, due to repeated trauma of these joints. Weight lifters commonly get arthritis in their shoulders and knees due to repetitive trauma to these joints. Tennis players often get arthritis in their dominant shoulder, whereas golfers commonly get it in their lower back. Continually moving these joints in the same way over time causes this arthritis, which can eventually lead to chronic trauma and then to degeneration of the joint.

A SELF-TEST FOR OSTEOARTHRITIS

The following symptoms are common to those suffering from osteoarthritis. Check the symptoms you have. If you have many of the symptoms below, check with your physician and a nutritional doctor for direction and guidance.

- I have early morning stiffness.
- I am stiff following periods of rest.
- My pain worsens with joint use.
- I have loss of joint function.
- My joints seem tender.
- My joints creak and crack with movement.
- My mobility is restricted.

Factory workers and construction workers also commonly develop osteoarthritis due to the repetitive nature of their work. For instance, a worker on an assembly line doing the same job over and over usually will develop arthritis in his fingers, whereas a carpet layer will develop it in his knees and hands.

A sheet-metal worker came as a patient to our office with swollen finger joints in both hands. He claimed that for the past thirty years he had been working with a nail gun that drives nails through metal. This worker is now on his way to overcoming arthritis, and you can be too.

Rheumatoid arthritis

Rheumatoid arthritis is different from osteoarthritis. It affects approximately 1.5 million American adults, striking women three times more often than men.[3] While osteoarthritis is age-related, rheumatoid arthritis is an autoimmune disease; with this condition the body is actually attacking itself. It not only affects the joints, but it also affects the entire body due to chronic inflammation. The joints affected are usually swollen, tender, warm to touch, and quite stiff.

Although many people associate rheumatoid arthritis with pain and swelling in the joints, it's actually a systemic disease that can affect other areas of the body as well. Fatigue, fever, and weight loss are very common symptoms during the early stages of the disease. Enlargement of the spleen and lymph nodes may also occur, as well as anemia, pericarditis, and lung disease.[4] Those with rheumatoid arthritis are also at higher risk for developing certain cancers, especially lymphoma.

A SELF-TEST FOR RHEUMATOID ARTHRITIS

If you are experiencing many of the following symptoms, consult with your physician.

- My age is between twenty-five and fifty.
- Pain and swelling in my joints developed within just a few weeks or months.
- The joints on both sides of my body are affected.
- My joints are swollen, red, and warm.
- I am experiencing general feelings of fatigue and sickness.
- I have lost weight.
- I often have a fever.
- I am stiff in the mornings.
- I have been experiencing major fatigue.

Let's stop right now and address the symptom of fatigue, most especially connected to rheumatoid arthritis. When you are tired and exhausted from pain, it seems impossible to maintain a positive outlook. You may feel discouraged, but God knows your circumstance. He will give you strength and rest. Take a moment right now to read aloud and meditate on these guidelines from Scripture for rest:

> He who dwells in the secret place of the Most High shall abide under the shadow of the Almighty. I will say of the Lord, "He is my refuge and my fortress; my God, in Him I will trust." Surely He shall deliver you from the snare of the fowler and from the perilous pestilence. He shall cover you with His feathers, and under His wings you shall take refuge; His truth shall be your shield and buckler. You shall not be afraid of the terror by night, nor of the arrow that flies by day, nor of the pestilence that walks in darkness, nor of the destruction that lays waste at noonday. A

> thousand may fall at your side, and ten thousand at your right hand; but it shall not come near you.
>
> —Psalm 91:1–7

Inflammation and Osteoarthritis

One of the marvels of your body is cartilage. God created the cartilage in your joints to be a remarkable shock absorber for your body. If you take care of your cartilage by drinking lots of water and losing weight, then you will be taking giant strides in successfully overcoming osteoarthritis.

There are many different types of joints in the human body, but there are three main classes—the fixed joints, the slightly moveable joints, and the highly moveable joints. The highly moveable joints are most commonly affected with osteoarthritis. These include the elbows, knees, shoulders, hips, fingers, toes, ankles, and wrists. Each of these joints is covered with articular cartilage. This cartilage is very smooth and shiny and is very similar in appearance to the cartilage on the drumstick of a chicken. It is bluish-white in color and is extremely smooth and slick. It is approximately eight times as slick as ice.

Cartilage serves as your body's shock absorber by cushioning the joints, and it prevents damage to the joint during different activities. It acts just like the air pocket in tennis shoes that allows us to walk on hard surfaces without any discomfort. Your cartilage serves just like this shock absorber. When it is healthy, we can engage in practically any sport or activity without pain. However, when the cartilage becomes thin and worn, we then develop pain with certain activities, which is analogous to wearing bargain tennis shoes, which have little to no cushioning, to play basketball on a hard gym floor.

Cartilage has no blood vessels in it; it depends on fluid exchange in order to be nourished. It is approximately 80 percent water, and the remainder of the cartilage is made up of collagen, proteoglycans, and chondrocytes.

Collagen is made up of amino acids that form protein chains. The collagen actually provides the strength and elasticity to the cartilage. It acts like reinforcement beams that hold the proteoglycans in place. Proteoglycans, on the other hand, are made of protein and sugar. They encircle the collagen fibers, forming a dense, water-loving, filler-like material in between the strong strands of collagen. They hold the collagen threads together, acting like a type of mortar. The cartilage gets both its shape and strength from the proteoglycans.

KNOW YOUR DISEASE: OSTEOARTHRITIS

- Caused by the wear and tear of cartilage
- Usually affects people after age forty
- Affects isolated joints, or joints on only one side of the body at first
- Causes discomfort in the joints but does not usually cause swelling; particularly affects the weight-bearing joints like the hips and knees
- Does not usually cause fatigue
- Causes brief morning stiffness

If the cells in your cartilage start dying due to toxicity, poor nutrition, or systemic disease process, then the cartilage is unable to be adequately repaired. Your cartilage framework then begins to splinter. The cartilage begins to crack and break off, and this leads to joint degeneration.

KNOW YOUR DISEASE: RHEUMATOID ARTHRITIS

- Is an autoimmune disease that often afflicts those from ages twenty-five to fifty
- Usually occurs in younger adults, but can attack children, even infants
- Usually affects joints on both sides of the body (e.g., both knees)
- Causes redness, warmth, and swelling of many joints and attacks many joints, often the small joints of the hands, feet, ankles, knees, and elbows
- Causes major fatigue of your whole body
- Causes prolonged morning stiffness

As the cartilage wears, enzymes are also leaked into the cartilage, which actually destroy more of the collagen and more of the proteoglycans. It then becomes a vicious cycle of joint destruction and increased joint pain. Eventually the cartilage becomes so thin and worn that it actually wears through, and the bone is exposed. When this occurs, it is very difficult to repair the cartilage. The body forms an inferior form of cartilage called fibrocartilage. This layer covers the bone. However, it only has a very short life span, so it is constantly being worn out. When this cartilage is finally gone, bone rubs upon bone, which causes severe pain. The bones also become extremely inflamed, and fluid from your cartilage leaking into the damaged bones causes even further damage.

As you can see, this is a vicious cycle that continues to get worse and worse. Therefore it is important to identify this disease early and to begin aggressive lifestyle and nutritional management as soon as possible. To keep your cartilage healthy, begin today to drink lots of water and eat right through proper nutrition.

Step 1: Drink water—lots of it

Water is extremely important in preventing osteoarthritis. Since cartilage is composed of approximately 80 percent water, I believe it is critically important to drink at least two quarts of water per day. Cartilage is similar to a sponge. The spongy cartilage soaks up synovial fluid when the joint is at rest. However, when pressure is placed on the joint, synovial fluid is squeezed out. The synovial fluid thus squeezes in and out of the cartilage with rest and activity. It is therefore critical to have sufficient water intake in order to have adequate synovial fluid.

As mentioned before, the proteoglycans of the cartilage are the primary portion of the cartilage that holds the water. With osteoarthritis the cartilage eventually dries out and thins. This then leads to cracking and further destruction of the cartilage.

RULE OF THUMB: H_2O

- Drink an 8- to 16-ounce glass immediately after waking up or half an hour before breakfast.
- Drink a glass fifteen to thirty minutes before meals or two hours after (except dinner). The more you drink, the fuller you will feel.
- With meals, drink only 4 to 8 ounces at room temperature.
- Avoid drinking large quantities after 7:00 p.m.

Step 2: Decrease inflammation through nutrition

As mentioned in a previous chapter, you can avoid certain foods that actually trigger inflammation, and this is especially important when it comes to the joint pain caused by inflammation for those suffering osteoarthritis. Additionally you can eat foods that will help strengthen and renew your cartilage. Let's explore how proper nutrition will help you win the battle against osteoarthritis.

Avoid foods with arachidonic acid. Arachidonic acid is a fatty acid that is found primarily in saturated fats and animal products.

These products include red meat, pork, egg yolks, poultry, and all dairy products except for nonfat dairy products. Arachidonic acid causes production of a dangerous form of prostaglandin, which actually promotes inflammation.

Avoid foods rich in omega-6 fatty acids. I believe dietary factors such as decreasing or eliminating dangerous fats and taking in the good fats on a daily basis are essential in controlling inflammation. As much as possible, then, avoid oils rich in omega-6 fatty acids, which include safflower, corn, and sunflower oils; margarine; and most other kinds of plant oils. Also avoid all fried foods.

Use extra-virgin olive oil and other foods high in monounsaturated fats. These include almonds, avocados, macadamia nuts, and canola oil. The Mediterranean diet that I outline in chapter 10, eaten by those living in the regions around the Mediterranean Sea, is rich in olive oil. In addition to its dietary and ceremonial uses, olive oil has historically been used medicinally. Beyond its natural healing properties, the Bible also instructs us to be anointed with oil for healing. (See James 5:14.) Accordingly I would encourage you to call upon your spiritual elders and have them anoint you with oil and pray for your healing. This will build your faith, strengthen your hope, and impart God's healing power upon you.

Eat foods rich in omega-3 fatty acids. EPA, which is an omega-3 fatty acid found primarily in fatty fish and marine plants, is very effective in reducing inflammation. Fatty fish include salmon, mackerel, herring, tuna, sardines, and trout. One should have at least three to five servings of fatty fish per week. If unable to eat these fish on a weekly basis, take omega-3 fatty acid supplements, approximately three capsules with each meal. You should also take digestive enzymes with these.

The Bible describes fish with fins and scales as being clean (Lev. 11:9). The Hebrews would often eat fish on the Sabbath. This could include all the fish mentioned above, which are rich in omega-3 fatty acids. Those clean foods are pure and healthy for you. God has provided healthy foods for you to eat and enjoy that will help your body heal and keep you in divine health.

REVELATIONS FROM ARTHRITIS RESEARCH

Epidemiological studies of Eskimos in Greenland have demonstrated the potential anti-inflammatory effects of omega-3 fatty acids, which are plentiful in their high-seafood diet. The Eskimos' prevalence of chronic inflammatory diseases is lower than that of inhabitants of Western countries.[5]

Inflammation and Rheumatoid Arthritis

As I stated above, rheumatoid arthritis affects approximately 1.5 million adults in America each year and is often seen as more difficult to treat than osteoarthritis. But good news has emerged both from research and faith. Studies have confirmed that many of the symptoms related to rheumatoid arthritis may be linked to food allergies. You can begin to feel better, reduce inflammation and pain, and begin experiencing God's healing power this very moment. How? Let me share with you some simple natural and spiritual steps.

Step 1: Eliminate certain foods.

Many people with rheumatoid arthritis have food allergies or sensitivities, and many common foods may trigger the symptoms of rheumatoid arthritis.

FOODS THAT TRIGGER RHEUMATOID ARTHRITIC REACTIONS

- Corn
- Wheat
- Pork
- Oats
- Rye
- Eggs
- Beef
- Coffee
- Oranges
- Grapefruit
- Milk and dairy products
- Nightshade plants, which include tomatoes, eggplant, potatoes, and bell peppers

To get to the bottom of your food allergies, you can perform a food elimination diet. Here's how you do it. First, for two weeks, stop eating the foods I have listed above. Then add one of the foods to your diet for a week. If you do not experience any increase in your rheumatoid arthritis symptoms during that week, then that food is probably safe for you to continue eating. If you have an increase in pain, swelling, redness, and warmth in your joints, then the food you added is possibly dangerous for you to eat. You may well be allergic or sensitive to it.

BEWARE OF THE NIGHTSHADE

Sensitivity to certain chemicals and foods you eat can trigger arthritis symptoms. In fact, nightshade plants are suspected to trigger the worst reactions.[6] Researchers have discovered that nightshade plants such as potatoes, tomatoes, eggplants, and peppers affect over one-third of those who suffer from rheumatoid arthritis. Already you have learned one simple thing you can do that may help relieve rheumatoid arthritis: decrease your intake of nightshade plants!

In the Bible, fasting serves spiritual purposes, but it can have natural benefits for your body. If you have been suffering from food allergies, fast for a few days with filtered or distilled water. You may also have white rice, since this is very hypoallergenic compared to most other foods.

I have also helped many of my arthritic patients who have food allergies with the NAET desensitization program. This therapy is used by physicians with extensive training in nutritional therapy. It is a natural, drugless, painless, and noninvasive method of elimination of allergies one at a time.[7]

EAT YOUR B_6

Researchers at Tufts University in Boston found that the B_6 levels in twenty-six rheumatoid arthritis patients were lower than the B_6 levels in healthy subjects. Foods rich in B_6 include brewer's yeast, brown rice, whole wheat, soybeans, rye, lentils, sunflower seeds, hazelnuts, alfalfa, salmon, wheat germ, tuna, bran, walnuts, peas, and beans.[8]

Step 2: Reduce intestinal inflammation through proper nutrition.

Reducing the inflammation of your digestive tract will help relieve some of the painful symptoms you may be experiencing. Proper absorption in your intestinal tract will insure that the nutrients you need for healing will reach your bones and joints. A healthy intestinal tract will greatly improve how you feel physically and will help reduce your arthritic symptoms. When you improve the condition of your digestive tract, then it can heal and maintain its normal permeability, thus allowing essential vitamins and minerals to reach your joints and bones with their healing properties.

The intestinal lining has one of the fastest growth rates of any tissue in the body other than the cornea. A completely new lining is formed every three to six days as the old cells slough off. You can help your irritated, inflamed intestine heal naturally through God-given substances, such as those listed below.

Ingest fish oil, evening primrose oil, and black currant oil. Essential fatty acids such as fish oil and evening primrose oil (one or two capsules three times a day with meals) and black currant oil (one capsule three times a day with meals) help maintain normal intestinal permeability.

TALK ABOUT TART!

Currants are mouth-puckering, which is why they are rarely eaten just out of your hand. Here are some palatable ways to prepare currants if you want to get their beneficial, healing effects without taking black currant oil capsules:

- Like cranberries, currants make a perfect sauce for livening up meat dishes. They're slightly sweeter than cranberries, however, so you'll want to add a combination of red, white, and black currants.
- Putting currants in fruit salads will add a tangy taste. For an even prettier plate, add a combination of red, white, and black currants.[9]

Maintain a high-fiber diet. A high-fiber diet will also improve intestinal permeability and help you overcome rheumatoid arthritis. There are many different forms of fiber, which include psyllium, oat bran, rice bran, ground flaxseeds, guar gum, and modified citrus pectin. Find your favorite form of fiber, and take it on a daily basis. I personally prefer fresh ground flaxseeds. However, you could also use over-the-counter psyllium products such as Perdiem Fiber, Metamucil, or oat bran.

If you have rheumatoid arthritis, see a nutritional doctor and have a comprehensive digestive stool analysis performed. To improve digestion, you may need to take betaine HCL and pepsin along with pancreatic enzymes. Thoroughly chew your food and mix it well with saliva; do not wash the food down with fluids. Again, a nutritional doctor will help to initiate a program to improve your digestion and intestinal permeability.

The Importance of Vitamins and Supplements

God's wonder substances for overcoming arthritis include vitamins and supplements. Of course, these natural substances are often found in nutritious foods; they may also be taken as supplements. God has created natural ways for our food and water to provide disease prevention and healing, but often our diets don't provide sufficient quantities of vital nutrients. That's why supplements are important. God gives us the responsibility to know how to care for our bodies naturally as well as how to apply His Word and pray spiritually for health.

Fighting osteoarthritis

Certain vitamins and supplements can help your body win its particular battle against arthritis. Let's take a look at the most prominent ones.

Vitamins C and E. When considering God's natural substances, we must first turn to His awesome vitamins C and E. Antioxidant vitamins such as vitamin C and vitamin E may decrease cartilage loss. It may also slow down progression of osteoarthritis.

Vitamin C and E work synergistically, and they both protect against the breakdown of cartilage. They may actually help form cartilage. Take 800 IU of natural vitamin E a day. You should also take at least 3,000 mg of vitamin C a day. I personally prefer the effervescent vitamin C known as Emergen-C.

DID YOU KNOW...?

Antioxidants like vitamins C and E are powerful agents that prevent oxidation caused by free radicals in our bodies. Free radicals are defective molecules that damage cells in our bodies.

God's wonder agents for helping our cells fight free radicals are antioxidants. Antioxidants are extremely important in strengthening our immune systems and helping our bodies overcome diseases like cancer, heart disease, and arthritis.

Multivitamins. A comprehensive multivitamin is necessary in order to have proper amounts of vitamins and minerals that are required for both the manufacture and maintenance of cartilage. The vitamins should contain adequate levels of the minerals zinc, copper, and boron, and also adequate levels of pantothenic acid, vitamin B_6, and vitamin A.

SAM-e. You might consider taking SAM-e, which is an amino acid that increases cartilage formation. While it is expensive, 200–400 mg of SAM-e two to three times a day may be effective in the manufacture of cartilage.

MSM. MSM (methylsulfanomethane) is another nutrient that may be effective in preventing or treating osteoarthritis. It contains high amounts of sulfur. Sulfur is an essential nutrient and is found in garlic, onions, and cabbage. Healthy cartilage needs adequate sulfur. I recommend 500 mg of MSM, two to three tablets, three times a day.

Glucosamine sulfate. In conventional medicine the common treatment of osteoarthritis is the use of nonsteroidal anti-inflammatory drugs (NSAIDs), such as ibuprofen and naproxen. NSAIDs work by blocking the production of certain prostaglandins that cause inflammation and pain.

While these anti-inflammatory medications help reduce some of your inflammation and pain, they also have many side effects that can be quite serious, including gastrointestinal bleeding (especially from stomach ulcers). Research has actually shown that long-term use of anti-inflammatory medications may impair healing of the joints. This may further damage the cartilage.

But God has provided a natural way for the treatment of inflammation and pain in your joints, known as glucosamine sulfate. In God's creation the lowly crab is linked to osteoarthritis through this God-created wonder substance found in the exoskeleton of arthropods like the crab. Studies have shown that patients can have as much as a 71 percent improvement using this awesome substance from God's natural created order.[10]

Glucosamine sulfate is a compound composed of glucose, glutamine (which is an amino acid), and sulfur. Glucosamine sulfate is used to manufacture proteoglycans. The proteoglycans are the mortar that holds the collagen together and retains the water in the cartilage. Due to the tremendous water content of the proteoglycans, the cartilage absorbs water like a sponge when pressure is released from a joint, and the cartilage squeezes that water out when pressure is put on the joint.

Glucosamine also may trigger the cells in your cartilage (chondrocytes) to produce more proteoglycans and collagen. In addition, glucosamine may help to repair damaged cartilage. Therefore, over time, supplementation with glucosamine sulfate will help to relieve pain from osteoarthritis. Glucosamine sulfate is also able to inhibit enzymes that break down the cartilage.

In studies that have compared glucosamine to ibuprofen, ibuprofen proved to be more effective in the first couple of weeks of therapy. After the second week on, however, the glucosamine group and the ibuprofen group were practically even in pain-relief effectiveness.[11]

And here's the real difference. Anti-inflammatory medications and pain relievers will mask the pain of osteoarthritis. As a result, you may feel that you can go out and exercise without any pain. However, in doing so, you may actually be doing more damage to the joint, since the anti-inflammatory or the pain medicine is only masking the pain.

Glucosamine sulfate, however, actually supplies the proteoglycans your cartilage needs, thus helping to repair the cartilage. More water is put into the cartilage. Therefore, after being on glucosamine sulfate for approximately a month, you should have minimal pain while exercising as compared to masked pain with an anti-inflammatory pain reliever. Glucosamine sulfate is a wonderful, God-created substance that can help your body fight back against osteoarthritis.

Anti-inflammatory supplements. As the joints in the body become progressively damaged by osteoarthritis, inflammation occurs. As mentioned earlier, inflammation is simply the body's natural response to damaged tissue. The inflammation then leads to warm, swollen, tender, and stiff joints. When the tissue is damaged, the body sends white blood cells to these areas of inflammation. The white blood cells produce leukotrienes and other products of inflammation, which thus cause more inflammation and create a vicious cycle.

If your osteoarthritis has reached the stage of chronic inflammation characterized by symptoms of swelling, stiffness, warmth, and pain, then you should immediately begin a diet of anti-inflammatory supplements.

Flaxseed oil is plant oil that helps to reduce inflammation. You may need to take extra zinc with flaxseed oil, so check with your nutritional doctor. I recommend 1 tablespoon of flaxseed oil two times a day, or five to seven capsules two times a day.

Quercetin and other bioflavonoids like quercetin enhance the absorption of vitamin C and are found in foods such as citrus fruits, green tea, and berries. You can also take quercetin in supplements. Normally, for every 500 mg of vitamin C, you should take at least 100 mg of quercetin or bioflavonoids.

Fighting rheumatoid arthritis

The typical treatments for rheumatoid arthritis are nonsteroidal, anti-inflammatory medications. These include naproxen and ibuprofen. However, this class of drugs can further damage your intestinal tract, leading to increased intestinal permeability or leaky gut. This leads to a worsening of food allergies, since our bodies absorb whole-food proteins.

In rheumatoid arthritis the contrast to osteoarthritis is that you need to address the issues of poor digestion, increased intestinal permeability, food allergies, and excessive inflammation. This needs to be done by a nutritional doctor. You may need an allergy desensitization diet, a comprehensive digestive stool analysis, and supplementation in order to heal your intestinal tract. However, here are some vitamin and mineral supplements that can get you started.

Multivitamins. Take a multivitamin that contains adequate amounts of B vitamins, minerals, and antioxidants, such as vitamins C and E.

Pantothenic acid and B-complex vitamins. A dose of 2 grams a day may significantly reduce morning stiffness and pain.

Vitamin C and bioflavonoids. These resources help reduce inflammation and histamine levels. I recommend 1,000 mg of vitamin C three times a day. Many people are allergic to vitamin C, since the majority of vitamin C comes from corn. Therefore, a patient with rheumatoid arthritis may need to be desensitized from corn in order to adequately absorb and utilize vitamin C. You can also find vitamin C buffered corn-free capsules in health food stores. Instead of deriving vitamin C from corn, these corn-free products derive vitamin C from such sources as the sago palm or beets.

Antioxidants. These are extremely important in overcoming rheumatoid arthritis. Take an antioxidant with a comprehensive antioxidant formula including vitamin C, beta-carotene, vitamin E, selenium, n-acetyl-cysteine, lipoic acid, grape seed or pine bark extract, and coenzyme Q_{10}. Grape seed extract and pine bark extract are particularly helpful with rheumatoid arthritis since they both help to relieve inflammation. You can find antioxidant capsules in health food stores.

I recommend 100 mg of grape seed or pine bark extract two times a day. The dose of vitamin C is 1,000 mg three times a day; vitamin E, 400 IU one to two times a day; beta-carotene, 25,000 units a day; selenium, 200 mg daily; n-acetyl-cysteine, 500 mg two times a day; lipoic acid, 100 mg daily; and coenzyme Q_{10}, 50 mg two times a day.

MSM. MSM is high in sulfur. Taking at least 500 mg three times a day may help to alleviate the pain and swelling of rheumatoid arthritis.

Proteolytic enzymes. These enzymes may help to decrease inflammation. They usually have to be taken in a dose of four to five tablets, three times a day, between meals. However, you should be under the care of a nutritional doctor in order to manage this appropriately. If you have ulcer disease or inflammation of the stomach or duodenum, you should not take proteolytic enzymes.

Bromelain. An enzyme that comes from pineapple, bromelain is similar to proteolytic enzymes. It also has a potent anti-inflammatory effect. The normal dose is 500 mg, one to two tablets, three times a day between meals.

Curcumin. This supplement comes from the yellow pigment of turmeric and has very strong anti-inflammatory properties. The normal dose of curcumin is 400 mg three times a day. It works especially well with bromelain when taken on an empty stomach.

Glucosamine sulfate. This natural supplement is still the standard approach in nutritional therapy for rheumatoid arthritis in a dose of 500–1000 mg three times a day. Glucosamine is a natural building block for the proteoglycans, one of the main components of cartilage.

Gamma oryzanol. This natural bran extract is made from rice bran. You should take 100 mg three times a day. Often taken as a natural muscle builder, gamma oryzanol also helps to heal the intestinal lining.

L-glutamine. Take L-glutamine, 500 mg, ten to thirty minutes prior to meals to help heal the intestinal lining. Also, taking the friendly bacteria, which is lactobacillus acidophilus and bifidus, helps to maintain a healthy intestinal environment in a dose of 3 billion colony-forming units per day.

Arthred. This molecular-weight hydrolyzed collagen is another very important nutrient for rebuilding cartilage. I recommend 1 heaping tablespoon of arthred a day.

Chondroitin sulfate. Chondroitin has been recommended in the past for treating both rheumatoid arthritis and osteoarthritis. However, it has very large molecules that are not well absorbed into the body when taken orally. Therefore I have recommended that patients take glucosamine sulfate instead of chondroitin sulfate.

Ginger. This herb has anti-inflammatory effects. A dose of approximately 4 grams of powdered ginger may be effective.

DHEA. I obtain a DHEA level on all patients with rheumatoid arthritis, and then I supplement them with DHEA. It is a hormone usually low in people who suffer from rheumatoid arthritis. A blood test by your nutritional doctor can help determine how much DHEA you may need.

Cetyl myristoleate. This fatty acid commonly found in beavers and sperm whales helps lubricate joints and reduce inflammation. A total dose of 1,000 mg a day under the supervision of a nutritional doctor is recommended.

Overcoming Arthritis With Exercise

While physical exercise may be painful for you at first, it is an essential ingredient in God's plan for overcoming arthritis. Exercise not only decreases the risk of developing heart disease, cancer, hypertension, diabetes, and osteoporosis, but it also decreases the risk of developing osteoarthritis. In other words, exercise helps prevent most degenerative diseases.

Do you already have osteoarthritis? Some exercises can actually worsen your condition, while others will greatly improve it. Do you have rheumatoid arthritis? Exercise can benefit you as well. Aquatic exercise can help both types of arthritis, because it is much easier on joints and muscles. Be sure to consult with your physician or physical therapist before starting any exercise program.

How does exercise help? It helps to improve the flow of synovial fluid into and out of the cartilage. This in turn keeps the cartilage healthy and moist and prevents the drying and thinning of the cartilage that is so often seen in osteoarthritis. It is extremely important for the synovial fluid to keep the cartilage moist and wet in order to prevent frictional forces that dry out the cartilage and cause wear and tear and thinning.

Exercise also helps you lose weight. One of the best preventive measures for osteoarthritis is reaching your ideal or normal body weight. As I said earlier, obesity and excess body weight are associated with increased stress on the weight-bearing joints, which will eventually trigger osteoarthritis.

I know that losing weight is more than just a physical issue. It's so important that you seek God's help to overcome any desire to overeat. Remember the promise of Scripture: "I can do all things through Christ who strengthens me" (Phil. 4:13).

When exercising, keep the following parameters in mind.

Drink adequate water. Again, adequate hydration and exercise are probably the two most important components in assuring adequate flow of the synovial fluid into and out of the cartilage, which is essential for osteoarthritis sufferers.

Maintain the range of motion of joints. The less a joint is used, the less range of motion you will maintain. An example of this is when a patient develops a painful shoulder and will not use the shoulder. He will not reach overhead or exercise the shoulder through a full range of motion. Within one to three weeks he may develop a frozen shoulder and be unable to extend his arm overhead or adequately rotate his shoulder. By not using the shoulder on a daily basis, he will actually lose the function of the shoulder. In other words, exercise maintains the flexibility of the joint. Avoidance of exercise can severely limit the normal range of motion of a joint.

Strengthen your tendons, ligaments, and muscles. Exercise strengthens the tendons, ligaments, and muscles that support the joint. This, in turn, adds more protection for the joint. Well-developed and well-toned muscles, tendons, and ligaments help to protect the joints by absorbing the majority of the force placed on the joints. Each time you exercise, you put pressure on the joints. The majority of the pressure is absorbed by the supporting structures, including the muscles, ligaments, and tendons.

Since cartilage has no blood vessels, the cartilage relies on an exchange of fluid through the synovial fluid in order to take in nutrients and eliminate waste products. Exercise encourages this process of taking in nutrients into the cartilage through the synovial fluid and expelling waste products or toxic material out of the cartilage.

Practice weight-bearing exercises. Weight-bearing exercises are some of the best forms of exercise for arthritis sufferers. However, if arthritis is severe, you should start with non-weight-bearing exercises and gradually work your way up. Weight-bearing exercises are exercises—such as walking, low-impact aerobics, and stair-stepping—where you are working against the force of gravity. These exercises help the bones grow stronger and thicker. However, this form of exercise is most effective for the lower part of the body, especially the ankles, knees, hips, and lower back, more so than the upper body.

Weight lifting and other isotonic types of exercises are also important in helping to build strong bones and muscles. You should lift light weights at very slow speeds and perform at least eight to twelve repetitions a set. To avoid injury, seek a certified personal trainer to instruct you on the proper techniques in lifting weights.

Practice aerobic exercise. Patients who have moderate to severe arthritis are often unable to walk sufficient distances to adequately work the muscles. Therefore for these patients I recommend alternative aerobic-type exercises. These include cycling, gliding machines such as the Precor machine, and water aerobics. These exercises take most of the strain off the joints while at the same time strengthening the supporting structures, tendons, and ligaments and stimulating the flow of the synovial fluid in the joints.

Prior to beginning an aerobic exercise program, you should be screened by your medical doctor in order to rule out significant cardiovascular disease. I recommend that my arthritis patients perform aerobic exercise three to four times a week for at least twenty minutes. Often arthritis patients are only able to start out at five minutes each time; gradually they can work up to twenty minutes by increasing the amount of exercise every week or two. I have seen so many of my patients who have begun to exercise on a regular basis improve to such an extent that I am able to decrease or eliminate their medications entirely.

FOUR IMPORTANT STEPS FOR OVERCOMING OSTEOARTHRITIS

- Drink 2–3 quarts of purified water daily for adequate hydration.
- Do regular aerobic exercise.
- Take glucosamine sulfate with adequate water consumption.
- Achieve ideal body weight.

Be sure to stretch. Stretching exercises are very important for both preventing arthritis and improving flexibility in arthritic joints. In starting an exercise program, it is best to warm up for five to ten minutes on a stationary bike, gliding machine, or treadmill. After you have adequately warmed your muscles up, then stretch anywhere from ten to twenty minutes. Stretching increases your flexibility, improves the range of motion of a joint, and makes you less prone to injury during weight-lifting exercises.

Follow a gentle program. After stretching, lift weights for approximately twenty to thirty minutes. I recommend weight machines rather than free weights since you would be less prone to injure yourself with the machines. After working out with weights, then perform aerobic exercise, such as cycling, gliding, stair-stepping, or walking on the treadmill for twenty minutes at your training heart rate.

After completing this, have a five-minute cooldown in which you walk at a slower speed. Then stretch slowly and hold the movement at the end of the stretch for approximately one to two seconds. If you develop pain in the joint, stop stretching in this manner. Count one, one thousand, two, one thousand, and then release the stretch. Perform anywhere from ten to twenty repetitions per movement. Some basic stretches include neck, back, knee, hip, and leg stretches.

Your prescription for overcoming arthritis includes regular exercise of your faith and your body. Don't give up and sit around nursing your pain. Take positive actions and think positive, faith-filled thoughts today. You can overcome arthritis when you take care of your body and exercise your faith boldly through prayer.

Action Steps

1. Do you suffer from osteoarthritis or rheumatoid arthritis?
2. How do you experience the effects of arthritis in your life?
3. If you have osteoarthritis, which of the following steps will you take?
   - Drink lots of water.
   - Avoid foods with arachidonic acid.
   - Avoid foods rich in omega-6 fatty acids. Use extra-virgin olive oil instead.
   - Eat foods rich in omega-3 fatty acids.
4. If you have rheumatoid arthritis, which of the following steps will you take?
   - Eliminate foods to which you are allergic.
   - Help your intestines heal using fish oil, evening primrose oil, or black currant oil.
   - Maintain a high-fiber diet.
5. Which of the following spiritual steps will you take?
   - Seek God's guidance in selecting the right foods to eat.
   - Ask God to help you avoid even shopping for foods to which you are allergic.
   - Pray for wisdom in caring for your body with proper nutrition.

Section II

INFLAMMATION REVERSAL BASICS

Chapter 5

HOW METABOLISM WORKS

Whether it's a nightly weather report showing the day's cloudscape or a montage of a busy street corner's ebb and flow of people, I love watching time-lapse videos. Observing hours, days, weeks, or months of time condensed into mere seconds fascinates me—and apparently it captivates others as well. Photographer John Novotny says that time-lapse photography has a way of affecting people intuitively: "They react to it with wonder, as if the act of making it surreal makes it more real, more beautiful. Of course, you can never beat the real thing, but...if done correctly, you can capture the essence of a place and portray it in a different way."[1]

My interest in this unique form originated with a documentary I saw years ago. It used time-lapse filming to capture the effects of the ocean on the coastline. I sat mesmerized as I watched waves pound away at the rocks, day after day, as tides flowed in and out. At first glance it appeared the water had no particular effect. Even after several years the coast essentially looked the same. Yet the producers proved that had their video been able to track thousands of years, I would have seen an entirely different landscape formed. By repeatedly and ceaselessly beating down the shoreline, the ocean actually wore down the rocks. Eventually the power of gradual erosion can reshape seemingly immovable structures.

In the same way that oceans can eat away at the shoreline,

repeat dieting—what many refer to as yo-yo dieting—has a similar effect on our bodies. The damage it causes wears down our metabolism. Generally, yo-yo diets decrease muscle mass and increase body fat. Even without dieting, after age thirty-five the average person loses between 5 and 7 pounds of muscle mass every ten years.[2] However, repeat dieters lose even more muscle mass. Even with many diets that result in weight loss, only approximately half of the pounds you lose are fat. The remainder is usually metabolically active muscle and water.

I cannot overemphasize how detrimental this is to gaining sustained control over your weight. Muscle is extremely valuable! Muscle cells burn about seventy times more calories than fat cells, which is why they are so crucial for maintaining weight loss.

Unfortunately, each time you hop on and off another diet, you typically lose valuable muscle and regain extra fat. Even worse, you gradually become fatter by dramatically lowering your metabolic rate. Studies show that with every decade of muscle loss, your metabolism also decreases by about 5 percent.[3] In essence, every time you drop another attempt at dieting, the more difficult you make the next one.

Before explaining how to halt this cycle and restore your metabolic system, we need to first look at how metabolism works.

Burn While You Rest

Metabolism is defined as the chemical processes continuously occurring in living cells or organisms that are essential for the maintenance of life.[4] It is the sum total of all chemical reactions in the body. Keep in mind that your tissues and organs never take a break. Your heart always pumps, your lungs always draw in breaths, and your liver never stops with its five hundred different functions, such as filtering the blood; removing toxins; processing fats, proteins, and carbohydrates; producing bile; and detoxifying chemicals, toxins, and metabolic waste. Your brain and nervous system, digestive system, immune system, hormones, bones, joints, muscles, and every tissue of your body all require energy.

These functions all contribute to your metabolic rate. Since it takes energy for your heart to beat, your lungs to breathe, and your organs to function properly, the metabolic rate is simply the rate at which you burn calories in a nonactive state. When considered over a twenty-four-hour period, this is called the basal metabolic rate (BMR), or resting metabolic rate. You typically burn about 75 percent of your calories during a state of rest. As I will discuss later, several things influence your metabolic rate, including stress level, muscle mass, eating behaviors, food choices, and activity level.

One of the biggest factors that affect the metabolic rate is skipping meals. When you do not eat for more than twelve hours, your metabolic rate goes down by about 40 percent. This sets you up for weight gain, which is compounded by consuming high-carbohydrate, high-fat foods, since your body will not burn as many calories in this lowered metabolic state. This is also why eating a healthy breakfast (literally breaking a "fast" through the night) is so essential. Individuals who eat breakfast are typically leaner than those who skip breakfast because this meal helps increase their metabolic rate.

As you might guess, body fat is not a metabolically active tissue. Muscle tissue, on the other hand, is extremely metabolically active. The more muscle you have, the higher your metabolic rate. The more fat, the slower your metabolic rate. Put another way, it takes far more energy to maintain a pound of muscle than a pound of fat. A good way to increase your metabolic rate is to increase your muscle mass and decrease your body fat.

ALL IN THE CALCULATIONS

Figuring out a ballpark basal metabolic rate (BMR) is easy.* There are more specific formulas for calculating your BMR, but to keep our discussion simple, I will share a general formula. There are three easy steps. First, simply multiply your weight in pounds by ten. Second, determine the number of calories you burn in a day by multiplying the number of minutes you exercise each day by four. Third, add this total to the first number.

For example, if you weigh 200 pounds and exercise thirty minutes a day, you would calculate your calories burned per day as follows:

- Body weight in pounds times ten (200 pounds x 10 = 2,000)
- Number of minutes exercised times four (30 minutes x 4 = 120)
- Add 2,000 to 120 = 2,120 calories burned per day

Remember that this is only a rough estimate of the metabolic rate; it does not apply to people who are metabolically compromised or have a depressed metabolic rate. Please refer to my book *Dr. Colbert's "I Can Do This" Diet* for more scientific formulas for BMR.

* When calculating BMR, it's important to realize that the typical male has significantly more muscle mass than a typical female, while women usually have a significantly higher amount of body fat than men. Therefore a one-size-fits-all BMR is not entirely accurate or realistic. The formula I discuss here is a very crude way to measure your BMR.

Easier Said Than Done

How many times have you heard someone make the simplistic statement "Losing weight isn't rocket science. All it takes is eating less and exercising more." Many of my obese patients would like to wring the necks of all the well-meaning but insensitive people who offer this as a word of "advice." As if these patients never tried that!

When it comes to weight loss, it is true that to shed pounds, we usually need to eat less and exercise more. However, what happens when doing these things doesn't work? What do you do when you have followed every diet and exercise program to the letter and still haven't seen results?

If this describes you, first let me remind you that you are not alone. As we explore the various reasons why people get stuck in their efforts to lose weight, you will see that many of these factors are reaching epidemic proportions. If you suffer from one or more of them, you are in the company of millions—and the club is growing.

Second, know that you may be metabolically compromised. All that means is that your metabolism is sluggish. Somehow—usually through chronic weight-loss diets and binge eating—it has become impaired to the point of barely working. This means your body isn't burning fuel the way it should be.

This can happen for a myriad of reasons, several of which you can find at www.thecandodiet.com. However, the overall result is that your body gets locked into storing fat instead of burning it. Sadly, many obese and metabolically compromised Americans are unaware of the factors that have contributed to their condition.

With that in mind, let's examine some of the major factors that can severely affect metabolic rate.

DR. COLBERT APPROVED—BREATHING TEST

A routine pulmonary lab test, called indirect calorimetry, can measure oxygen consumption, carbon dioxide production, and respiratory exchange rate. This test is the best way to measure your BMR, providing accurate and useful information in providing a detailed picture of the body's metabolic processes at rest.[5]

Chronic Stress Lowers Metabolic Rate

Our bodies are designed to secrete two stress hormones when we are stressed: epinephrine and cortisol. A "fight or flight" hormone, epinephrine works immediately by racing through our bodies when triggered by such stressors as an emergency, running late for an appointment, or an argument with a spouse. When our bodies are unable to fight or flee, we become like rush-hour commuters stuck in bumper-to-bumper traffic on the interstate—we are left literally stewing in our own stress juices. Epinephrine revs up the stress response by raising our blood pressure and increasing both our heart rate and our breathing. When the perceived stress is over, the epinephrine level typically drops back to normal.

On the other hand, cortisol works more slowly, giving us stamina to cope with long-term stress. However, when the stress response becomes stuck as a result of long-term stress, the ongoing elevation of cortisol causes the body to continually release sugar from glycogen into the bloodstream. Glycogen is simply stored sugar, generally held in the liver and muscles. When glycogen is released into the bloodstream, it causes insulin levels to rise, which in turn lowers the blood sugar. Low blood sugar causes more cortisol to be released, leading to weight gain. Excessive insulin also causes the body to store fat in adipose tissue, while also preventing the body from releasing fat from the tissues, even during exercise. In other words, stress programs us for fat storage and contributes significantly to insulin resistance. Through this process such chronic stress lowers the metabolic rate.

Elevated cortisol levels can also cause the body to burn muscle tissue as fuel. Cortisol is a catabolic hormone, which means it causes the body to break down muscle to produce energy, leading to an even lower metabolic rate. As any weight lifter knows, muscle tissue is pricey fuel; we sacrifice our metabolic rate when we burn muscle tissue as fuel. Cortisol is the only hormone that increases as we age.

Certain foods and beverages will raise cortisol levels, including everyday items such as caffeinated beverages and coffee. In fact, drinking two cups of coffee raises your cortisol levels by approximately 30 percent within a single hour. I am not recommending that you stop drinking coffee, since it does have health benefits. However, I recommend a maximum of two cups a day.

Eating excessive amounts of sugar, white bread, and other high-glycemic foods without the proper ratio of protein, fats, and fiber can cause hypoglycemic episodes. These are bouts with low blood sugar that also raise cortisol levels. Whenever your blood sugar drops, your body is naturally signaled to increase cortisol production. Another way this can happen is through food allergies and sensitivities and by skipping meals and snack times.

Your Gender Plays a Part

Women typically have a higher percentage of body fat and lower metabolic rate than men. There is currently no consensus on a specific "healthy" range of body fat percentage, and ranges vary according to age. However, most studies indicate a good goal for women is to keep your body fat under 30 percent (for women, obese is defined as a body fat percentage—not BMI—greater than 33 percent; 31–33 percent is borderline). For men, that goal is less than 20 percent (for men, obese is defined as greater than 25 percent; 21–25 percent is borderline).[6]

By design women have a lower metabolic rate than men because they typically carry an additional 7 to 8 percent of fat, even at a healthy weight. Add to this the fact that a woman's metabolic rate declines at the rate of approximately 5 percent per decade of her life, starting at age twenty.

Inactivity and Muscle Loss

Sedentary individuals as they age have a significant loss of muscle mass. Earlier I stated that adults naturally lose 5 to 7 pounds of muscle every ten years after age thirty-five; as you might guess, inactivity further accelerates this process. The less active we are, the more body fat we keep—and, naturally, the more muscle we lose. By age sixty most people have lost about 28 pounds of muscle and have replaced most of that with much more fat.

I have found this to be especially true among women. I check body fat measurements on all my weight-loss patients and have commonly encountered women with 50 percent body fat or more. Yet it is extremely rare to find this among male patients. Most high-body-fat cases stem from a combination of gender and lack of exercise, plus metabolic compromise.

Obviously women have a disadvantage by carrying a higher percentage of body fat; generally they do not lose weight as fast as men. Because of this, it is even more important to educate them about the effects exercise has on metabolism, as well as help them understand the unique challenges they face. A sedentary lifestyle compounds the situation and increases their chances of obesity, laying a foundation for developing type 2 diabetes.

SIT OR GET FIT?

Obese people sit down an average of 152 minutes more each day than more slender individuals.[7]

Could Your Medication Be to Blame?

A common side effect of certain medications is weight gain. These medications include birth control pills, hormone replacement therapy, prednisone and other steroids, various antidepressants, antipsychotic medications, lithium, insulin and insulin-stimulating medications, cholesterol-lowering medications, some anticonvulsant medications, some antihistamines, and certain blood pressure pills, such as beta-blockers. Ironically, many physicians treat diseases caused by obesity such as hypertension, diabetes, depression, and elevated cholesterol with the very medications that lower the metabolic rate and result in more weight gain. That is why I typically use vitamins, supplements, and other nutrients in conjunction with a sensible eating plan to treat obesity-associated problems rather than just medications.

A Problem of Thyroid

Though often overlooked in the weight-loss equation, a low or sluggish thyroid can also cause a decreased metabolic rate. I have seen hundreds of cases in which patients reached the end of their rope after adhering to every diet under the sun but never losing weight, only to discover that their thyroid was inhibiting their progress. Thyroid blood tests should be checked regularly to ensure that the thyroid is functioning normally.

Although men can develop thyroid disease as well, the overwhelming majority of those suffering from thyroid issues are women. An estimated 13 million American women have some kind of thyroid dysfunction.[8] The sad part is that many of them do not even know it and struggle with weight loss (along with other issues) their entire lives. I discuss the reasons why I believe this goes undiagnosed in *Dr. Colbert's "I Can Do This" Diet*. Researchers say that about 10 percent of younger women and 20 percent of women over age fifty regularly experience mild thyroid problems that impact their weight, attitude, and overall health.[9]

The two main hormones produced by the thyroid gland are thyroxine (T4) and triiodothyronine (T3). Most of the thyroid hormone in the body, or around 80 percent, is T4. T3 is the active form of thyroid hormone and is several times stronger than T4. It is also very important for weight loss. Eighty percent of the T3 in our bodies comes from the conversion of T4 to T3 in such organs and tissues as the kidneys, liver, and muscle. Both of these thyroid hormones gradually decline with age. Yet many obese people may show signs of a sluggish thyroid. I believe one of the main reasons for this is because some are poor converters of T4 to T3. After seeing hundreds of obese people in my practice struggle to convert T4 to T3, I have identified the following reasons for their poor conversion: chronic unremitting stress, taking certain medications (birth control, estrogen and

HRT, beta-blockers, chemotherapy, theophylline, lithium, and Dilantin), eating certain foods (soy, excessive consumption of raw cruciferous vegetables, low-fat diets, low-carb diets, and low-protein diets), and excessive alcohol intake.

Half the Equation

Every overweight individual has a reason for his or her overweight condition. Yet sadly, most who have struggled unsuccessfully with diets over the long haul never discover the underlying reasons for their inability to shed pounds. In this chapter I have touched on many of these various causes as they relate to metabolic rate, ranging from skipping meals to chronic dieting to chronic stress to aging to medications to low thyroid. In doing so, I have tried to help you understand the many ways your metabolic rate can be affected—which you now know directly influences maintaining weight loss and blood sugar levels.

This is only half the equation, however. Revealing how metabolism works is essential for understanding how to lose pounds and keep them off. Just as important is knowing the solution: developing a low-glycemic lifestyle. With that in mind, in the next chapter I will look at how to raise your metabolic rate and keep off those pounds for good.

Action Steps

1. Would you guess that you have a high metabolism or a low metabolism?
2. Why?
3. Which of the following factors could be contributing to a lower-than-optimum metabolism for you?
   - Chronic stress
   - Gender
   - Inactivity and muscle loss
   - Medication
   - Thyroid issues
4. Calculate your basal metabolic rate according to the formula given in this chapter.

Chapter 6

THE STARCH AND SUGAR TRAP

A lot of people think eating fat makes you fat. It's actually the way your body *stores* fat that makes you gain weight. Overconsumption of carbohydrates and sugars stimulates your body's production of insulin—which is the body's fat storage hormone. Insulin lowers blood sugar levels when they are too high. However, elevated insulin levels also cause the body to store fat.

For example, when you eat foods that are high in carbohydrates, such as breads, pasta, potatoes, corn, and rice, the carbohydrates are broken down to glucose, which is absorbed into the bloodstream. If insulin levels are elevated, the carbohydrates are more likely to be converted to fat by the liver and then stored away in fat cells.

Easier On Than Off

If you consume a lot of starch and sugar on a frequent basis, your insulin levels will remain high. If insulin levels remain high, your fat is, figuratively speaking, locked into your fat cells. This makes it very easy to gain weight and extremely difficult to lose weight. Elevated insulin levels usually prevent the body from burning stored body fat for energy. Most obese patients cannot break out of this vicious cycle because they are constantly craving starchy, sugary foods throughout the day, which keeps the insulin levels elevated and prevents the body from burning these stored fats.

The average person can store about 300–400 grams of

carbohydrates in the muscles and about 90 grams in the liver. The stored carbohydrates are actually a stored form of glucose called glycogen. However, once the body storehouses are filled in the liver and muscles, any excess carbohydrates are then usually converted into fat and stored in fatty tissues. When you skip meals or go more than four to five hours without eating, the blood sugar usually decreases, unleashing a ravenous appetite.

FIVE SNACK DUDS

1. Cookies (even if they're fat free, watch out for those calories and sugar)
2. Granola bars (some pass the test, but most are loaded with sugar)
3. Chips and nachos (fat, fat, fat...the bad kind too)
4. Cakes and pastries (tons of calories, lots of sugar and fat, and zero nutrition)
5. Crackers (although few are OK, many are loaded with butter or oil)

Exercise may not help you if you don't eat right. If you eat refined carbohydrates throughout the day, much of the excess carbohydrates will be converted to fat. The high insulin levels also make it more difficult for the body not to release a significant amount of its stored fat. Therefore you can work out for hours at a gym and still not lose fat because you are eating high amounts of carbohydrates and sugar throughout the day. Your body usually will store excess carbohydrates as fat and make it difficult to release any fat that is already stored.

To make matters even worse, when you consume sugar or starches frequently, especially cake, candy, cookies, fruit juices, ice cream, or processed white flour, you may develop low blood sugar within a few hours after eating and unleash a ravenous appetite for more sugar and starch. This raises your blood sugar and your insulin levels, programming you for even more fat storage and preventing you from burning stored fat when you exercise. How frustrating this can be for the uninformed patient! Symptoms of low blood sugar include spaciness, shakiness, irritability, extreme fatigue, headache, sweatiness, racing heart, extreme hunger, or an extreme craving for sweets or starches.

Caught in a Trap

This creates a vicious cycle. If you don't eat something sweet or starchy every few hours, you may develop the symptoms of low blood sugar. This is a very important point. You can turn this entire situation around very easily by taking a very simple step: avoid sugar and refined starches.

By avoiding sweets, starches, snack foods, junk foods, or high-carbohydrate foods, you can lower your insulin levels and turn off the main trigger that is telling the body to store fat and preventing the body from releasing fat.

When the brain doesn't get enough glucose, you will get cravings. The brain requires a constant supply of glucose. When too much insulin is secreted, such as when you consume a snack that is high in sugar (i.e., a doughnut, a Coke, or cookies), the pancreas then responds by secreting enough insulin to lower the sugar. Often too much insulin is secreted, which lowers the sugar too much, thus causing low blood sugar. Since the brain is not getting the glucose it requires, the low blood sugar creates sugar and carbohydrate cravings, extreme hunger, mood swings, fatigue, and problems concentrating. The brain releases different hormones to increase one's appetite. These signals cause the individual to reach for a sugar or starch "fix" in order to raise the blood sugar the fastest, which will then be able to supply the brain with adequate glucose.

RULE OF THUMB: BREADS

The more processed and refined bread is, the less fiber it contains—and, ultimately, the less filling it is. Look for brands that contain at least 3 grams of fiber per slice. I also recommend double-fiber breads and sprouted breads.

The Power of Glucagon

Glucagon is a hormone that works totally opposite than insulin works. Insulin is a fat-storing hormone, whereas glucagon is a fat-releasing hormone. In other words, glucagon will actually enable the body to release stored body fat from the fatty tissues and will permit your muscle tissues to burn your fat as the preferred fuel source instead of blood sugar.

How do you release this powerful substance into your body? It's easy. The release of glucagon is stimulated by eating a correct amount of protein in a meal along with the proper balance of fats and carbohydrates. We will look at this in greater detail later on.

When the insulin levels are high in the body, the level of glucagon is low. When glucagon is high, then insulin is low. When you eat a lot of sugar and starch, you raise your insulin levels and lower your glucagon, thus preventing fat from being released to be used as fuel. By simply stabilizing your blood sugar and lowering your insulin levels, you can keep your glucagon levels elevated, which enables your body to burn off the extra fat. Thus you'll begin to realize a more energetic, slimmer you! Eating your protein first helps boost glucagon levels, or you can eat a salad with sliced chicken, turkey, or fish.

Should You Count Calories?

Many people still say, "Why not count calories? A calorie is a calorie." Most people believe that since fat has 9 calories per gram and carbohydrates have only 4 calories per gram, then eating a gram of fat is much more fattening than eating a gram of carbohydrate. But the hormonal effects of fat are not nearly as dramatic as the hormonal effects of carbohydrates and sugars.

Fats will not raise insulin levels, which programs the body to store fat. However, sugars and starches will trigger dramatic releases of insulin, which is the most powerful fat-storing hormone. So don't count calories. Instead be aware of how your body works. Keep in mind the powerful hormonal effects that sugars and starches have on both insulin, the fat-storing hormone, and on glucagon, the fat-releasing hormone.

The Bible says, "Surely, in vain the net is spread in the sight of any bird" (Prov. 1:17). That means you cannot capture a prey if it understands what's happening. By understanding this powerful truth about how your body actually works, you can avoid the trap of high blood sugar, of high insulin levels, of being overweight or obese, and even of diabetes. Now that you know, the power is in your hands!

Glycemic Index 101

The glycemic index was created in the early 1980s to track how quickly insulin levels shot up in individuals after they consumed carbohydrates. While studying individuals with type 2 diabetes, researchers found that certain carbohydrates increased blood sugar levels and insulin levels, while other carbohydrates did not. They tested hundreds of different foods to determine their glycemic index value. Because their methods and findings have proven so reliable, they are the standard by which we measure the internal processing of foods.

The glycemic index assigns a numeric value to how rapidly the blood sugar rises after consuming a food that contains carbohydrates. Sugars and carbohydrates that are digested rapidly, such as white bread, white rice, and instant potatoes, rapidly increase blood sugar. These are high-glycemic foods and have a glycemic index of 70 or higher. On the other hand, if foods containing carbohydrates are digested slowly and therefore release sugars gradually into the bloodstream, they have a glycemic index value of 55 or lower. These foods include most vegetables and fruits, beans, peas, lentils, sweet potatoes, and the like.

Because these foods cause the blood sugar to rise more slowly, blood sugar levels are stabilized for a longer period of time. Low-glycemic foods also cause satiety hormones to be released in the small intestines, which satisfies you for longer periods of time.

In truth, there is nothing fancy about the glycemic index. One of the most important factors that can determine a food's glycemic index value is to what degree the food has been processed. Generally speaking, the more highly a food is processed, the higher its glycemic index value; the more natural a food, the lower its value.

THE GLYCEMIC INDEX

- Low-glycemic foods: 55 or less
- Medium-glycemic foods: 56 to 69
- High-glycemic foods: 70 or above

The Glycemic Load

Almost twenty years after the glycemic index was created, researchers at Harvard University developed a new way of classifying foods that took into account not only the glycemic index value of a food but also the quantity of carbohydrates that particular food contains. This is called the glycemic load. It serves as a guide as to how much of a particular carbohydrate or food we should eat.

For a while nutritionists scratched their heads over patients who wanted to lose weight and were eating low-glycemic foods yet weren't shedding many pounds. Some actually gained weight. Through the glycemic load they discovered that overconsuming many low-glycemic foods can actually lead to weight gain. Not surprisingly many patients were eating as many low-glycemic foods as they wanted, simply because they had been told that foods with a low value promoted weight loss. They needed to know the whole story, which is how the glycemic load balances the picture.

DR. COLBERT APPROVED—GOING LOW GLYCEMIC

A recent study of the Dutch population found that by lowering the glycemic index value of overall food intake by an average of ten points, participants decreased their CRP levels by 29 percent. Participants who continued on a low-glycemic diet also had higher levels of good cholesterol, improved insulin sensitivity, and reduced chronic inflammation—all of which indicated a decrease in risk of metabolic syndrome and cardiovascular disease.[1]

A food's glycemic load is determined by multiplying the glycemic index value by the quantity of carbohydrates a serving contains (in grams) and then dividing that number by 100. The actual formula looks like this:

- (Glycemic Index Value x Carb Grams per Serving) ÷ 100 = Glycemic Load

To show you how important the glycemic load is, let me offer some examples. Some wheat pastas have a low glycemic index value, which makes many dieters think they're automatically a key to losing weight. However, if a serving size of that wheat pasta is too large, it may sabotage your weight-loss efforts. Despite a low glycemic index value, the pasta's glycemic load is high. Another example is white potatoes, which have a glycemic load double that of yams. On the other end of the scale, watermelon has a high glycemic index value but a very low glycemic load, which makes it OK to eat in a larger quantity.

Don't worry, though. You will not have to calculate the glycemic load for every item you eat. By understanding this concept, you can identify which low-glycemic foods can cause trouble if you eat too much of them. These include low-glycemic breads, low-glycemic rice, sweet potatoes, yams, low-glycemic pasta, low-glycemic cereals, and so forth. As a general rule, any large quantity of a low-glycemic "starchy" food will usually have a high glycemic load.

GLYCEMIC INDEX VALUES OF COMMON FOODS[2]

Food*	Glycemic Index Value
Asparagus	15
Broccoli	15
Celery	15
Cucumber	15
Green beans	15
Low-fat yogurt (artificially sweetened)	14
Peppers (all varieties)	15
Spinach	15
Zucchini	15
Cherries	22
Milk (skim)	32
Apples	38
Spaghetti (whole wheat)	37
All-Bran cereal	42

GLYCEMIC INDEX VALUES OF COMMON FOODS (continued)	
Food*	**Glycemic Index Value**
Orange juice	52
Bananas	54
Potato (sweet)	54
Rice (brown)	55
Muesli	56
Whole-wheat bread	69
Watermelon	72
Doughnut	76
Rice cakes	82
Corn flakes	83
Baguette (French bread)	95
Parsnips	97
Dates	103

** To look up the glycemic index values of other foods not listed above, go to www.thecandodiet.com.*

The amount of fiber in your food, the amount of fat, how much sugar is in the carbohydrates, and proteins all determine the glycemic index score of what you eat.

Three Types of Sugar

Three main types of simple sugars (called monosaccharides) make up all carbohydrates. These include:

- Glucose
- Fructose
- Galactose

Glucose is found in breads, cereals, starches, pasta, and grains. Fructose is found in fruits. Galactose is found in dairy products. Plain sugar, or sucrose, is a disaccharide and consists of glucose and fructose joined.

The liver rapidly absorbs these simple sugars. However, only glucose can be released directly back into the bloodstream. Fructose and galactose must first be converted to glucose in the liver to gain entrance into the bloodstream. Thus they are released at a much slower rate. Fructose, found primarily in fruits, has a low glycemic index compared to glucose and galactose.

HIGH-FRUCTOSE CORN SYRUP: SUGAR IN DISGUISE

If you have diabetes, your doctor has undoubtedly told you how important it is to limit the amount of sugar in your diet. Although you know you need to choose your foods carefully, food manufacturers can be sneaky. One ingredient to be extremely wary of is the presence of one of sugar's many aliases: high-fructose corn syrup (HFCS).

HFCS is a blend of glucose and fructose. Glucose is the form of sugar in your blood that you monitor as a diabetic. Fructose is the primary carbohydrate in most fruits. Well, if it's from fruit, it's healthy, right? Not exactly. It is true that it's OK to consume small amounts of fructose because your body metabolizes it differently. As a result, it does not trigger your body's appetite control center. However, consuming large amounts sets you up for increasing belly fat and a fatty liver, insulin resistance, and eventually diabetes.

Since HFCS is common in thousands of commercial food and drink products, I highly recommend that you stick to the outer aisles at the grocery store, where you will find fresh produce, whole grains, and lean meats. Avoid the center aisles, where the highly processed foods, boxed convenience items, and sugar-laden treats live. Follow this commonsense approach, and you will be well on your way to avoiding the risk of consuming the "stealth" sugar that hides inside many packaged, processed products. Many researchers believe that America's excessive intake of HFCS is responsible for our diabetes epidemic.

How bad is it? HFCS represents 40 percent of caloric sweeteners added to foods and beverages and—until the advent in recent years of pure-sugar versions of various soft drinks—was the only sweetener of soft drinks in the United States.[3] The average American consumes about 60 pounds a year of HFCS. "So what?" you shrug. You may take a more serious outlook when you realize that the liver metabolizes fructose into fat more readily than it does glucose. This means that consuming HFCS can lead to a non-alcoholic fatty liver, which usually precedes insulin resistance and type 2 diabetes.

Almost every product on the grocery shelves today contains both nutritional information and a list of ingredients. Too many people complain that they don't understand these labels or that it takes too much time to read them. If you are battling diabetes or prediabetes, it will be well worth your time to get educated. And when it comes to HFCS, here is a simple rule to follow: If HFCS is one of the first ingredients on the label, don't eat or drink it.

Here is a sampling of foods high in HFCS:

- Soft drinks
- Popsicles
- Pancake syrup
- Frozen yogurt
- Breakfast cereals
- Canned fruits
- Fruit-flavored yogurt
- Ketchup and barbecue sauce
- Pasta sauces in jars and cans
- Fruit drinks that are not 100 percent fruit

Other Glycemic Foods

Fiber is a form of carbohydrate that is not absorbed. However, it does slow down the rate of absorption of other carbohydrates. Thus the higher the fiber content of the carbohydrate or starch, the more slowly it will be absorbed and enter the bloodstream.

Most fruits are high in fiber and have a low glycemic value.

The exceptions are bananas, raisins, dates, and other dried fruits. Almost all vegetables are high in fiber and low glycemic except for potatoes, carrots, corn, and beets, which have a high glycemic value.

In the next chapter we will discuss in more detail the best foods to eat for overall good health and especially if you want to lose weight. The right carbohydrates balanced with the proper portions of proteins and fats will create a much lower glycemic effect on your body and interrupt the vicious cycle of weight gain.

Action Steps

1. What are the top five problem foods that you crave?
2. What are three foods with a low glycemic index or low glycemic load that you can eat more often?
3. What five fruits or vegetables will you begin to incorporate into your diet?
4. In what ways do you need God's help to change your eating habits?

Chapter 7

RIGHT KNOWLEDGE FOR EATING RIGHT

God skillfully designed your body as an incredible, living creation that will operate at peak efficiency and health when it is supplied with proper nutrition. In a previous chapter we looked at many of the reasons Americans are obese. Now I want us to take a look at the powerful nutritional foundation that will help you to discover a healthier, happier, more attractive you. And once we've settled on the foundations of good food to eat, I'll provide you in the next section with a specific diet to follow to reverse inflammation's disruption in your body once and for all.

Choosing the Right Carbohydrates

Certain carbohydrates are critical for good health. When combined with the correct portions of fats and proteins, good carbs give you energy, calm your mood, keep you full and satisfied by turning off hunger, and assist in weight loss. They also help you to enjoy meals and snacks, enable you to handle stress better, allow you to sleep more soundly, improve your bowel function, and give you an overall feeling of well-being.

However, as with so many things in the land of excess, most Americans have fallen in love with the wrong kind of carbs. They see their waistlines getting wider and wider as a result of eating too much sugar, starch, bread, and pasta, and they think the answer is to swear off all carbohydrates. The problem is, high-protein diets are often hard to maintain for long, and in some cases they have damaging effects on health. The answer isn't a no-carb diet but one rich in the *right* kinds of carbohydrates.

The National Institutes of Health recommends that 45 to 65 percent of daily energy intake for adults come from carbohydrates, with 20 to 35 percent of energy coming from fats and only 10 to 35 percent from proteins.[1] The American Diabetes Association also recommends 45 to 60 grams of carbohydrates in each meal, preferably from healthy whole grains.

I believe this is too many carbohydrates and too much grain. I believe excessive carbohydrates and grains—especially wheat and corn products—are one of the main reasons for our obesity epidemic. I typically recommend about 50 to 55 percent of daily calories come from low-glycemic carbohydrates, 15 to 20 percent from plant and lean animal proteins, and 25 to 30 percent from healthy fats.

Because wheat and corn can trigger exaggerated blood sugar responses, I have my patients give up all wheat and corn products for a season or until they reduce their belly or body fat. Even if breads at the supermarket are called whole-grain breads, they still contain amylopectin A, which usually spikes blood sugar, programming the body for fat storage and weight gain. Therefore if my patients request bread, I recommend that they have small amounts of millet bread in the morning or at lunch. It contains no wheat. However, if weight loss stalls, I have my patients stop eating millet bread. Once a person reaches his goal waist measurement or weight, if he can practice moderation, I have him add back small servings of wheat and corn for breakfast or lunch, but not dinner.

GOOD FRUITS

A Brazilian study found that women who ate three small apples or pears a day lost more weight on a low-calorie diet than those who didn't add fruit to their diet. Because of the high fiber in these fruits, those fruit-eating females aiso ate fewer calories.[2]

The Tortoise and the Hare

So, how can a person know which are the right carbs to choose? Many people are familiar with the old story about the tortoise and the hare. The hare races ahead but fails to reach the finish line, while the slow but steady tortoise eventually passes him and wins the race. When it comes to how your body processes carbohydrates, the race that takes place within you is reminiscent of this classic fable. I've used these familiar characters to identify two main types of carbohydrates we will talk about in this chapter: low-glycemic "tortoise carbs" and high-glycemic "hare carbs."

Unfortunately most of the carbohydrates overweight and obese people consume are high-glycemic "hare carbs," which cause the blood sugar to rise rapidly. As I have already alluded to, this starts a chain of events that traps people in a fat-storage mode and prevents them from losing weight. The underlying cycle of hare carbs is obvious enough: the faster you absorb the carbs, the higher your insulin level rises, the more weight you gain, and the more diseases you develop. You become literally programmed for weight gain.

When it comes to weight-loss success, "tortoise carbs" are the long-term winners. These are the carbohydrates that slowly raise the blood sugar and enable you to lose weight and prevent or reverse diseases. These low-glycemic tortoise carbs can be broken down into the following groups:

- Vegetables (except potatoes)
- Fruits (except bananas and dried fruits)

- Starches, such as millet bread, brown rice pasta, steel-cut oatmeal, sweet potatoes, new potatoes, brown rice, and wild rice, in small quantities (minimize these starches; some patients have to eliminate them altogether)
- Dairy products, such as skim milk; low-fat, low-sugar yogurt; kefir; and low-fat cottage cheese (minimize these products)
- Legumes, such as beans, peas, lentils, hummus, and peanuts (I recommend 1–4 cups of these starches a day, but start with small servings; you may also need Beano, an enzyme that helps you digest beans and minimize gas)
- Nuts and seeds (raw; a handful a day)

Even though most of these tortoise carbohydrates are healthy, it's still possible to choose the wrong types of starches and dairy or overeat low-glycemic starches, such as millet bread and brown rice pasta. For this reason, and because there are other ways carbohydrates stall weight-loss efforts, it's important to incorporate the glycemic index and glycemic load principles I discussed in the previous chapter.

Is It a Hare or a Tortoise?

The faster your body digests a carbohydrate, the faster it raises your blood sugar—and the higher the glycemic index value of that carb. This is what makes a carb a hare rather than a tortoise. Yet how exactly can you differentiate between the two? Here are a few traits that will help distinguish between a tortoise and a hare.

Fat content. With the exception of seeds, nuts, and dairy, most tortoise carbohydrates are low in fat. Fats are not an inherent evil, as some diets claim. But consuming highly processed, high-fat carbohydrates will sabotage your weight-loss efforts.

Fiber content. Generally a higher fiber content of a food slows down the absorption of sugar, making the carb a tortoise. Beans, peas, and lentils are high in fiber.

Form of starch. Certain starches, such as potatoes, bread, pasta, and white rice, contain amylopectin, which is a complex carbohydrate that the body rapidly absorbs and that usually raises your blood sugar. However, beans, peas, legumes, and sweet potatoes contain another complex carb called amylose, which is digested more slowly and raises the blood sugar in a slower fashion. Caution is needed with whole-wheat products, as I have discussed. Almost all corn products are considered hare carbohydrates (with a high glycemic index value). Exceptions are corn on the cob and frozen corn, because they are digested more slowly and gradually raise the blood sugar.

Ripeness. The riper the fruit, the faster it is absorbed. For instance, brown, spotted bananas raise blood sugar much faster than regular yellow bananas since they have a higher sugar content.

Cooking. Most brown rice pasta can be either a tortoise carbohydrate or a hare carbohydrate, depending on how you cook it. If you cook it al dente, still leaving it firm, it is typically a tortoise carbohydrate and has a low glycemic index value. Also, thicker pasta noodles generally have a lower glycemic index value than thinner types of pasta (angel hair, thin spaghetti, etc.). Again, I don't recommend any wheat pasta products, even whole grain, since they have a higher glycemic load than many other carbohydrates.

Milling type. A finely ground grain is a hare carbohydrate and has a higher glycemic index value than coarsely ground grain, which has a higher fiber content and thus is a tortoise.

Protein content. The higher the protein content of a food, the more it helps prevent a rapid rise in blood sugar and makes the food more likely to be lower glycemic. Thus it is a tortoise carbohydrate.

DR. COLBERT APPROVED—PGX FIBER

PGX, short for PolyGlycoPlex, is a unique blend of highly viscous fibers that act synergistically to create a much higher level of viscosity than the individual fibers alone. PGX absorbs hundreds of times its weight in water over one to two hours and expands in the digestive tract, creating a thick gelatinous material. It creates a feeling of fullness, stabilizes blood sugar and insulin levels, and stabilizes appetite hormones.

PGX lowers blood sugar after eating by about 20 percent and lowers insulin secretion by about 40 percent. Researchers have found that higher doses of PGX can decrease appetite significantly. PGX works similar to gastric banding and has fewer gastrointestinal side effects than other viscous dietary fibers. However, start slowly, or you may develop gas.

To aid in weight loss, I recommend starting with two or three capsules of PGX fiber with 16 ounces of water before every meal and gradually increasing the dose if needed. This usually prevents you from overeating and enables you to feel satisfied sooner. (See appendix.)

Please Pass the Unprocessed, Unrefined, Complex Carbs

Here's another way to put it: if we are ever going to reclaim our good health, we must get off of our refined carbohydrate kick. We eat far too many highly processed, overly refined, devitalized carbohydrates. We make selections that pack our GI tract with dead, devitalized substances that harm, not heal, our bodies. Here are a few examples of refined carbohydrates you should limit or avoid altogether:

- White bread
- Pasta

- Sugars such as sucrose and high-fructose corn syrup
- Cornstarch
- French fries
- Most breakfast cereals
- Cookies
- Cakes
- Bagels
- Pretzels

Eating large amounts of refined grains and sugars creates more inflammation in the body. Refined carbohydrates, such as white sugar and white flour as well as corn and potatoes, cause a rapid rise in blood sugar, which causes more insulin to be released from the pancreas. Excess insulin creates more oxidative stress, which, in turn, creates more inflammation.

To counter this vicious cycle, choose unrefined carbohydrates found in whole grains, fruits, and vegetables. Sadly only 9 to 32 percent of Americans consume five daily servings of vegetables and fruit as recommended by the federal government.[3] And many who do choose potatoes and corn as vegetables, which can actually create more inflammation.

Unrefined carbohydrates generally have a lower glycemic index, meaning they don't cause the blood sugar to rise rapidly. Forty percent of your total caloric intake should be from unrefined carbohydrates, such as whole grains, fruits (not fruit juice), and vegetables.

FLOUR POWER

When I was growing up, my mother had to carefully store flour in airtight containers, and she had to use it up very quickly. That was because flour, even the processed varieties, had a relatively short shelf life. If not stored carefully and used quickly, my mother would open up a container and look inside to find that it was full of bugs and unusable.

That seems like a very unpleasant experience. But has it ever happened to you? Probably not. Do you know why? Because the flour we purchase in the grocery store today has been so overly processed that it no longer contains any nourishment for bugs. Food companies are happy because they have extended the shelf life of flour and grains to an almost unlimited amount of time. Those who bake with flour have been happy as well because they no longer have to wonder if bugs have ruined their flour.

So, if everyone is happy, what could be wrong? Well, stop for a minute to consider that if the processed flour in your pantry no longer nourishes a bug, neither will it nourish you. Many of today's breads, cakes, rolls, tortillas, buns, cookies, and pies are made from flour that has virtually no nutritional value at all. It is almost as dead as the bag of plaster in your garage.

When our daily dietary choices are made up of dead foods, not only are our bodies being denied the vital nutrients they need, but they are also forced to deal with the impact of digesting and eliminating dead foods. And we wonder why we are battling an epidemic of disease in this country. Just imagine what it might do to your body to eat that bag of plaster from your garage every day. It's a mental picture that can make you start thinking about whether you are choosing living foods or dead foods!

Remember, you are alive and your body is a living organism, which is why it requires living foods.

The Power of Protein

Proteins and amino acids are the building blocks for the body. They are used to repair and maintain tissues such as muscles, connective tissue, skin, hair, bone matrix, and even nails. If you do not have adequate protein, you will not be able to adequately maintain these tissues I just listed, as well as enzymes, hormones, and your immune system. As a result, you will age faster and eventually develop disease.

But in the same way too many low-glycemic carbs can sabotage your weight-loss goals, so can too much protein have a negative effect on your well-being. Studies have shown that men with diets high in red meat have an increased risk of prostate cancer, and it is typically a more aggressive form of prostate cancer. However, men who eat fish three times a week have approximately half the risk of developing prostate cancer compared to men who rarely eat fish. Also, frying or grilling meat, chicken, or fish so that it is charred or well done is also associated with an increased risk of cancer.

In 2002 the National Institutes of Health advised that protein should make up 15 to 35 percent of a person's daily consumption of energy or total calories. I believe that anything more than 35 percent of our daily calories as protein is simply too much. I tell my patients to get approximately 15 to 20 percent of their daily calories from protein, but I recommend only 10 percent or less of our calories should come from animal protein. This usually translates into 3 ounces of animal protein once or twice a day for women and 3 to 6 ounces of animal protein once or twice a day for men. Men should limit red meat to only 12 ounces a week. I also strongly believe in consuming some protein with each meal and snack; however, we don't need animal protein with each meal.

Beans and a small amount of brown rice (the size of a tennis ball) is a complete protein. This helps to create the correct fuel mixture that keeps your appetite controlled, your energy up, and your blood sugar and insulin levels in check—all while your metabolism continues to burn off those extra pounds.

Free-range or organic lean chicken and turkey; organic or omega-3 eggs; wild-caught, low-mercury fish; and organic low-fat dairy are the best choices of animal proteins. These meats are free of hormones and antibiotics that can be harmful to the body. Also avoid or limit high-fat junk meats such as hot dogs, bologna, salami, pepperoni, and bacon, which are loaded with salt, nitrates, and nitrites. Nitrates and nitrites are associated with an increased risk of certain cancers.

Organic legumes, whole grains, and nuts are the best plant proteins. Vegetarians are able to combine plant proteins with their regular meals to have a high-quality protein. For example, by combining whole-grain rice and beans, you can form complete proteins. Soy, however, is an exception and is already considered a complete protein.

The potential problem with combining two starches to make a complete protein is that it is easy to slow down or entirely stop your weight loss if your portions are too big. If you can keep this in mind, however, there is no reason you should not enjoy the added benefits and flavors of these proteins. Black bean soup or lentil soup and a small amount of wild rice is a complete protein and very filling—and yes, you will most likely start losing weight if you regularly consume it.

IT'S ALL ABOUT FIBER

Since only 5 percent of Americans consume an adequate amount of daily fiber, women hoping to lose weight should concentrate more on getting enough fiber rather than following through with low-carb, low-fat, or high-protein diets. This was confirmed by a study of more than 4,500 people, which also discovered that women on a low-fiber, high-fat diet have an increased risk of being overweight or obese.[4]

Plant-based protein powder is also a good way to add protein to your meals and snacks. But you should consume soy products with caution. Many scientists now believe that overconsuming soy may do more harm than good. High consumption of isoflavones, which are the estrogen-like plant chemicals contained in soy, may stimulate the production of breast cancer cells. It may also increase the chances of developing serious reproductive, thyroid, and liver problems.[5]

Besides this, most soy products are processed and have a low biological value compared to other proteins—meaning the body doesn't use them very efficiently. This includes two of the most commonly consumed soy products, soy milk and soy protein. These products can interfere with thyroid function and lower the metabolic rate, making it more difficult to lose weight.

I recommend cutting back on soy products if you desire to lose weight. And let me emphasize this: the final word on soy is not yet in. Even the soy skeptics say the bottom line is to opt for natural forms of soy rather than chemically altered or genetically modified (GM) forms. Because it remains a somewhat controversial protein, my advice is to proceed with caution; do not eat or drink soy products every day, but if you must consume soy, do it only a few times a week.

The Fat Truth

For decades physicians, nutritionists, dietitians, and other health authorities have blamed fats for every diet-related problem under the sun: the obesity epidemic, elevated cholesterol, and heart disease. It's as if someone devised a master plan to take a single "truth" and transform an entire nation's dietary mind-set. The premise: all fats make you fat.

As a result, people flocked like lemmings to anything labeled "low-fat" or "no fat." Everyone started going on low-fat diets, cooking from low-fat cookbooks, and eating low-fat crackers, low-fat chips, low-fat ice cream, and low-fat cookies. Americans decreased their consumption of fat from 45 percent of daily caloric intake in the mid-1960s to 38 percent in the 1980s to approximately 35 percent of calories in the mid-1990s.[6] One problem, though: we kept on gaining weight.

In fact, obesity has skyrocketed in this country to unparalleled proportions while the average weight of Americans has steadily increased too. If fats are supposed to make you fat, then why has cutting back on them made Americans fatter? Something doesn't add up. Here's the truth: fats don't necessarily make you fat. There are bad fats that put on weight, but there are also good fats that enable you to lose weight. The good fats help prevent heart disease, lower triglycerides, and ward off a multitude of diseases. The bottom line is that too much of any fat—good or bad—will make you fat.

Still, fats are vital for good health. Among their many roles they provide fuel for your cells. A fatty cell membrane, composed primarily of polyunsaturated and saturated fats, surrounds each of the trillions of cells in your body. Saturated fats provide a rigid support for the cell membrane. Polyunsaturated fats add flexibility to the cell membranes and allow the transfer of nutrients inside cells and waste products to pass to the outside. These cell membranes need a proper balance of both.

Likewise we need a balance of fats in our diet to help with the absorption of fat-soluble vitamins, including vitamins A, D, E, and K. And we need fats to produce hormones that regulate inflammation, blood clotting, and muscle contraction. Approximately 60 percent of your brain is composed of fat. You need cholesterol to make brain cells, and most cholesterol comes from saturated fats. Fats make up the coverings that surround and protect nerves. They help to satisfy hunger for extended periods.

Types of Fats

Fats can be broken down into two main types: saturated and unsaturated. Within the unsaturated fats category are three smaller groupings, which are omega-6 fats, omega-9 fats, and omega-3 fats.

Omega-3 and omega-6 fats are polyunsaturated fats, while omega-9 fats are monounsaturated fats. Only two fats within these subcategories are required for health: linoleic acid, an omega-6 fatty acid, and alpha-linolenic acid, an omega-3 fatty acid. Our bodies are capable of producing all other types of fats by consuming these two. That leaves omega-9 fats left out in the rain, since they are considered nonessential.

Since all this may leave you scratching your head, I have categorized fats into three main categories: bad fats, good fats, and fats that can be good or bad, depending on the amount ingested.

Bad Fats

Trans fats

These are man-made fats, such as those present in margarine, shortening, most commercially baked foods, many deep-fried foods, many commercial peanut butters, and processed foods such as crackers, cookies, cakes, pies, and breads. The problem with trans fats is that they are synthetic and toxic. They are inflammatory fats that raise cholesterol, form plaque in the arteries, and increase the risk of obesity, heart disease, type 2 diabetes, and cancer.

How bad are trans fats? Open up a tub of margarine and set it outside. Typically even insects won't go near it. So how in the world did we wind up putting this substance in the majority of our foods? Good question. After being developed in Germany and mass-produced in England, trans fats came to America in 1911 with the introduction of Crisco. To boost sales, the company gave away cookbooks in which every recipe required this hydrogenated shortening.[7] By the advent of World War II—with butter in short supply—trans fats became ingrained in our culture. Processed food companies had the perfect fat. It was cheap, it wouldn't spoil, and it had an extremely long shelf life.

My, how the times have changed. In January 2007 the US

Food and Drug Administration (FDA) almost banned Crisco. Rather than fold up shop, though, the product's maker agreed to reformulate its shortening to contain zero trans fats per serving.[8] This fell more in line with the government's general recommendation to either not eat trans fats or only in very small quantities. The reasons go beyond adding pounds. By consuming trans fats, your cells and cell membranes become hydrogenated or partially hydrogenated, growing rigid and stiff.

Researchers found out that women who consumed the most trans fats—about 3 percent of daily energy, or about 7 grams of fat—over a fourteen-year period were twice as likely to develop heart disease than those who ate the least amounts.[9] Overall, experts agree that each gram of trans fat consumed increases the risk of heart disease by approximately 20 percent. In addition, trans fats further obesity risks by increasing insulin resistance and the size of fat cells, which in turn enables them to store more fat.

FOODS THAT OFTEN HAVE TRANS FATS

- Fast foods
- Packaged foods
- Frozen foods
- Candy and cookies
- Baked goods
- Chips and crackers
- Toppings, dips, and condiments
- Soups
- Margarine and butter
- Breakfast foods

The public is slowly catching on to the dangers. Beginning in 2006, the FDA mandated labeling of all foods containing trans fats. Fortunately many fast-food restaurants and processed food companies dropped their use. But that does not mean we can celebrate. When Dunkin' Donuts shed trans fats in 2007, they switched to a blend of palm, soybean, and cottonseed oils[10] (still not a health food). Check fast-food offerings and others on store shelves. Learn to read labels, and avoid foods containing hydrogenated or partially hydrogenated oils or trans fats.

READ YOUR FOOD LABELS

Since foods can still contain up to 0.5 grams of trans fats per serving while being labeled as having zero trans fats, the best way to avoid consuming trans fats unawares is to look for the words *partially hydrogenated* or *shortening* on the label or ingredient list. If you find either, don't eat the product!

Refined polyunsaturated fats

This is another type of bad fat that causes weight gain. The majority of Americans consume excessive amounts. These fats are found in most salad dressings and commercial vegetable oils, such as sunflower, safflower, corn, cottonseed, or soybean oil. These omega-6 fats have been refined and heated to high temperatures. Thus they are typically high in dangerous lipid peroxides, which trigger inflammation. These fats are also associated with weight gain because of their tendency to increase insulin resistance.

MISLEADING LABELS

On January 1, 2006, all packaged foods sold in the United States began to list trans fat content on their nutrition labels. But under FDA regulations, "if the serving contains less than 0.5 gram [of trans fat], the content, when declared, shall be expressed as zero."[11] That means you could eat several cookies, each with 0.4 grams of trans fat, and end up eating several grams of trans fats—even though the label says zero!

Deep-fried foods

Deep-fried foods, such as french fries, onion rings, fried chicken, deep-fried fish, fried corn or potato chips, and hush puppies, are loaded with inflammatory fats. Imagine taking a sponge, dropping it in water, and wringing all of the water out. That is similar to what you are doing when you toss french fries, onion rings, or chicken into a deep fryer. That food is literally soaking up the grease and fat. Instead of wringing it out of a sponge, you put it in your mouth. In the process your body is being programmed to store fat. Parents who regularly feed their children french fries, deep-fried chicken, and fried chicken strips are unknowingly setting up their children for a lifelong struggle with obesity.

Fats That May Be Good or Bad

Some fats can be good or bad, depending on the amount ingested. These include saturated fats and unrefined omega-6 fats, which are polyunsaturated fats.

Saturated fats

Are these good or bad? It depends on the type and amount consumed. Saturated fats are found primarily in animal products, including meat such as beef, pork, lamb, and poultry. More precisely, they lie in animal fat—the visible fat around a piece of steak or marbled fat mixed with meat, which makes prime rib and rib eye steaks so juicy. Finally, saturated fats are found in poultry skins; dairy products such as butter, cream, and cheese; and a few vegetable oils—palm oil, palm kernel oil, and coconut oil.

Thousands of studies prove that excessive intake of saturated fats is associated with an increase in LDL cholesterol (the bad kind) and increased risk of atherosclerosis and cardiovascular disease.

Many people are unaware of the many types of saturated fats. The short-chain variety is present in coconut oil and palm kernel oil, both of which are excellent sources of fuel for the body and easily digestible. These fatty acids are healthier and less likely to elevate cholesterol levels (unless consumed in excess). Coconut oil also contains lauric acid, which helps immune system function and is present in breast milk.

The next type includes medium-chain triglycerides (MCTs). These are also found in coconut oil and palm kernel oil. These fats are digested and utilized differently than other saturated fats. They first go to the liver and are rapidly converted to energy. Athletes use these fats quite frequently; they produce immediate energy, and the body typically does not store them as fat. MCTs also help increase the metabolic rate. Yet be aware MCTs can be stored as fat, especially with too many calories and a lack of exercise.

The worst types of saturated fats are the long-chain saturated fats, especially in such fatty cuts as most hamburger meat, ribs, rib eye, prime rib, sausage, and bacon. All are associated with raising LDL cholesterol. Long-chain saturated fats are present in all meat and high-fat dairy products such as butter and cheese.

Saturated fats should make up approximately 5 to 10 percent of your food intake. However, if you have elevated levels of cholesterol, the American Heart Association's Nutrition Committee recommends no more than 7 percent of your daily calories come from saturated fat.[12] When you consistently consume more than 10 percent of total calories as saturated fat, you increase your risk of high cholesterol, atherosclerosis, insulin resistance, and weight gain.

Cutting back

So, how do you lower your intake? Choose extra-lean cuts of meat and low-fat or nonfat dairy products, remove poultry skins, trim off all visible fats, and limit red meat to two or three times a week (a maximum of 18 ounces a week, although I recommend no more than 12). I recommend more turkey and chicken breast, which are typically low in saturated fats—provided they are free range and organic. I also like fish, low in mercury, but be careful to avoid farm-raised varieties. Fish with low mercury levels according to the FDA include anchovies, butterfish, cod, flatfish, haddock, hake, herring, jacksmelt, mackerel, perch (ocean), pollack, salmon (canned), salmon (fresh/frozen), sardine, tilapia, trout, tuna (especially tongol tuna), whitefish, and whiting. Women should limit portion sizes of these proteins to 2 to 6 ounces per meal while men should aim for between 3 and 8 ounces.

This may seem like a small amount, especially to men accustomed to huge steaks. No matter how much you love steak, though, it is loaded with saturated fats that lock you into obesity, often via insulin resistance. Remember that free-range, grass-fed, or organically fed animals—buffalo, bison, or elk—typically have much less saturated fat than grain-fed animals.

Omega-6 fats

We all need small amounts of unrefined omega-6 fats on a daily basis for good health. For example, everyone requires linoleic acid, but most people take in excessive amounts, often in the form of salad dressings and refined oils (corn, soy, sunflower, safflower oil, cottonseed oil). Many processed foods, fast foods, and restaurant foods are extremely high in refined omega-6 fatty acids. The recommended ratio of omega-6 fatty acids to omega-3 fatty acids should be approximately four to one. Currently most Americans consume about a twenty-to-one ratio![13] Omega-3 fats suppress inflammation; omega-6 fats promote it.

Instead of refined omega-6 fats, choose small amounts of expeller- or cold-pressed oils: extra-virgin olive oil, high oleic safflower, and sunflower oil, which are high in monounsaturated fats. Healthy sources of omega-6 fats include most seeds and nuts. Although seeds and nuts are high in fat, they are also high in fiber, which is filling, satisfying, and prevents some fat absorption. Keep in mind that an excessive consumption of even good omega-6 fats can cause weight gain and promote inflammation, which is at the root of most chronic diseases, including obesity and type 2 diabetes. As always, the key is moderation.

Healthy Fats

GLA

Gamma linolenic acid (GLA) is produced in the body from linoleic acid (LA). Think of GLA as a "super LA." It is a beneficial fatty acid that helps to decrease inflammation. Oils that contain GLA include borage, evening primrose, and black currant seed oil. Unfortunately GLA is not found in most foods. Even though LA is an essential fatty acid, many individuals are unable to convert LA to GLA and are thus at a higher risk of developing inflammation, impaired immune response, allergies, and insulin resistance. This also means that the risk of weight gain and fat storage increases due to their bodies' inability to produce adequate amounts of GLA.

Most people who naturally produce GLA are young and healthy. This is because the body's ability to convert LA to GLA is impaired by excessive amounts of stress; the intake of trans fats, saturated fats, and omega-6 fats; and aging.

Omega-3 fats

Without getting into too many details, it is important to explain a bit more about omega-3 fats, since they are often automatically associated with fish. There are three types: alpha-linolenic acid (ALA), found in flaxseeds and flaxseed oil; eicosapentaenoic acid (EPA), found in cold-water fish; and docosahexaenoic acid (DHA), found in cold-water fish and some algae. Approximately 99 percent of Americans are deficient in these healthy fats.

Unfortunately many individuals are unable to produce EPA and DHA from ALA because of impairments in the enzyme making this conversion, usually from stress, aging, and excessive intake of trans, saturated, and omega-6 fats. Therefore, even if you are eating a lot of flaxseed oil and flaxseeds, you still may not have adequate amounts of EPA and DHA.

Omega-3 fats, particularly EPA and DHA, have many benefits. They decrease inflammation, lower triglycerides, assist in preventing and treating heart disease, support the immune system, and prompt the release of stored fat. The best sources of omega-3 are fatty fish, such as salmon, mackerel, herring, and sardines. Quality fish oil supplements are good alternatives.

A diet with sufficient amounts of omega-3s will usually prevent and may eventually reverse insulin resistance. These fats help the body shed abdominal weight. Good fats in the form of fatty fish or fish oil capsules are a must for anyone wanting to lose weight in this region. And omega-3 fats also decrease the risk of developing diabetes.

I mentioned earlier the benefits of choosing free-range, grass-fed, or organically fed animals. Animals that are typically grain fed include cows, pigs, and even chickens. Their meat usually contains a very low concentration of omega-3 fatty acids and significantly higher amounts of omega-6 fatty acids. Grain-fed meat is also typically high in saturated fats. However, free-range or grass-fed animals typically have much higher concentrations of omega-3 fats in their tissues and lower levels of omega-6 and saturated fats.

DR. COLBERT APPROVED—SALAD DRESSING

Treat your health to this delicious salad dressing made with beneficial fats.

- 1 cup extra-virgin olive oil (cold pressed)
- ¼ cup balsamic vinegar
- 2 fresh basil leaves, chopped
- 1 small clove fresh garlic, crushed

Store in a salad dressing carafe. Shake well before using.

Note: Create your own dressing recipes with olive oil and your favorite spices.

Monounsaturated fats

These are also good fats. Certain Mediterranean diets consume up to 40 percent of their daily calories from monounsaturated fats, primarily in the form of olive oil. In what became known as the Seven Countries Study, Ancel Keys, PhD, and other researchers studied more than twelve thousand men between the ages of forty and fifty from 1958 to 1964.

Keys discovered that those in the Mediterranean groups had the lowest mortality rates from all causes. Greek men had the lowest mortality rate overall and the lowest rate of heart disease. Finnish men had the highest rate of heart disease. They consumed almost 40 percent of calories from fats, with more than 50 percent coming from saturated fats. Among other things, the study proved that olive oil and other monounsaturated fats are extremely healthy fats.[14]

Monounsaturated fats are in the omega-9 category and are considered nonessential, since the body can make them from other fats. Regardless, monounsaturated fats are extremely healthy and are anti-inflammatory, helping lower LDL cholesterol without decreasing good HDL cholesterol. They also help to support the immune system and aid weight loss.

Foods high in monounsaturated fats include olives, olive oil, avocados, almonds, hazelnuts, pecans, cashews, macadamia nuts, peanuts, peanut oil, Brazilian nuts, sesame seeds, sunflower seeds, pumpkin seeds, and canola oil. Since most fats are inflammatory and promote insulin resistance, the root cause of diabetes, I have my diabetic patients choose mainly omega-3 fats and monounsaturated fats, which are both anti-inflammatory.

FATS THAT MAKE YOU SKINNY

A study from Brigham and Women's Hospital in Boston reveals why, for weight loss, a Mediterranean-style diet using olive oil trumps a traditional low-fat diet. Those on the latter limited fat intake to 20 percent of calories, while those on the Mediterranean diet could obtain 35 percent from olive oil, nuts, and other monounsaturated fats. After six months both groups lost weight. Yet after eighteen months only 20 percent of those on the low-fat diet stuck with it, and most regained weight. The majority of those on the Mediterranean diet not only stayed on it, but they also kept their pounds off.[15]

The Big Fat Problem

The majority of Americans consume approximately one-third of their total calories from fats. Even though this is a fairly safe amount, Americans continue to gain weight and suffer from an epidemic of being overweight and obese and of suffering from prediabetes and type 2 diabetes. For this reason I recommend approximately 25 to 30 percent of your total calorie intake as fats (making sure to choose good fats) in order to improve insulin resistance, decrease inflammation, and lose weight. I cannot stress enough the importance of both the type of fats and the ratio of fats consumed.

I suggest about 10 to 20 percent of your fat intake be monounsaturated fats and 5 to 10 percent polyunsaturated fats, with a four-to-one ratio of omega-6 to omega-3 fats. In other words, if 2.5 grams of your fats are omega-3 fats, consume 7.5 grams of omega-6 fats, with GLA being the best form of omega-6 fats. Finally, no more than 5 to 10 percent of fat intake should be saturated fats. I recommend avoiding all trans fats, fried foods, and refined omega-6 fats, such as most regular salad dressings.

Whenever I explain fats to patients, I say they simply need an oil change. You would not think of driving year after year without changing your car's oil because eventually you would ruin the engine. Your body is no different. You need the proper balance of healthy oils in your body for healthy cells, tissues, and organs.

Fats are not evil; however, inflammatory fats such as trans fats, fried foods, omega-6 fats, and saturated fats make one more prone to develop insulin resistance and eventually prediabetes and diabetes. You can use the right proportion and amount of good fats to help you lose weight. Now go get an oil change.

Action Steps

1. How will you add more good carbohydrates into your diet?
2. How will you add more protein to your diet?
3. What foods do you need to eliminate from your diet?
4. Pray and ask God to help you choose foods that will allow your body to function at its best.

Section III

YOUR INFLAMMATION REVERSAL GAME PLAN

Chapter 8

BEATING INFLAMMATION THE NATURAL WAY

Would you like a supernatural guarantee for success? Here it is: The Bible says to commit your plans to the Lord. "Commit your works to the LORD, and your thoughts will be established" (Prov. 16:3). So I want to encourage you to study the plan outlined in this chapter and then commit it to the Lord for the strength and willpower to follow through.

God is greater than any bondage you may have. And He promises to help you succeed, not with your own power, but by asking for His. He is so faithful. When you ask Him for help, He promises never to fail you or leave you struggling all alone. The Word of God says, "For He Himself has said, 'I will never leave you nor forsake you'" (Heb. 13:5). What a powerful promise!

In this chapter we will look at the special eating plan I've created that will help you reverse inflammation as well as create a path to healthy, consistent weight loss. But first, a word of caution. As I have said before, the number on the scale is not the best measure of weight loss. Make sure you keep the right focus. Instead of focusing on how much you weigh, focus on eating right. When you eliminate sugar, sweets, excessive carbohydrates, bad fats, wheat, and corn from your diet, you will most likely begin to lose weight. Best of all, you will eliminate chronic inflammation and set yourself on a path toward lifelong health, free from disease and ailment.

A Deadly By-Product of the Western Diet: Inflammation

One of the biggest problems with our modern high-fat, highly processed, high-sugar, high-grain (such as wheat and corn), high-sodium diets is that it has thrown off the balance in our bodies between inflammatory and anti-inflammatory chemicals called *prostaglandins*. As we already learned, inflammation is normally a good thing that works to repair an injury or fight off infection in the body. It puts the immune system on high alert to attack invading bacteria or viruses to rid our body of these intruders, or, in the case of an injury, it rushes white blood cells to the cut, scrape, sprain, or broken bone to remove the damaged cells, splint the injury, or attack infections to facilitate healing.

This is the good side of inflammation and an extremely important function of the immune system's small agents. When our bodies are in such an emergency, there is a complicated process through which more pro-inflammatory prostaglandins are created than anti-inflammatory ones, and the immune system responds to the sounding of this alarm. When the crisis is over, the balance swings in the anti-inflammatory direction and eventually balances out again.

If you look at this process in a grossly simplified sense, you will see that prostaglandins are produced from the foods we eat in an ongoing cycle, and each of the foods we eat has either a pro-inflammatory tendency or an anti-inflammatory one. Fatty acids are at the center of this. Omega-6 fatty acids are "friendly" to the creation of pro-inflammatory prostaglandins, and omega-3 fatty acids are "friendly" to the creation of anti-inflammatory prostaglandins. A more natural, Mediterranean-type diet will have a balance of pro- and anti-inflammatory-friendly foods; however, our modern high-fat, high-sodium, high-sugar, highly processed Western diet throws that balance off in favor of the production of pro-inflammatory prostaglandins.

Experts tell us that our typical US diet has doubled the amount of omega-6 fatty acids we consume since 1940 as we have shifted more and more away from fruits and vegetables to grain-based foods and the oils produced from them. In fact, we eat about twenty times more omega-6s than we do the anti-inflammatory omega-3s. Most of the animals we obtain food from today are also grain fed, so most of our meats, eggs, and dairy products are higher in omega-6s than they were a century ago. Also, as most of the fish in our stores are now farm raised, they are fed a diet of cereal grains instead of the algae and smaller fish they would live on in the wild, so even our fish are more sources of omega-6s than they used to be. Noting all of this, it is not hard to see why diseases caused by chronic systemic inflammation have grown to be such a problem in the Western world today.

Furthermore, essential fatty acids (EFAs) such as omega-3 and omega-6 cannot be manufactured in the body and must be consumed either through diet or supplements. EFAs help the body repair and create new cells. In addition to reducing inflammation, omega-3 fatty acids can actually create special roadblocks in the body, making it harder for cancer cells to migrate from a primary tumor to start new colonies. Cancers that remain localized in one place are much easier to treat than those that metastasize (spread throughout the body).[1]

Because of the high omega-6 content of our diets, our bodies find more material for pro- than anti-inflammatory prostaglandins. Over time the natural, ongoing creation of prostaglandins will tip the balance toward systemic inflammation as more pro-inflammatory prostaglandins are produced than anti-inflammatory ones. Despite the absence of an actual emergency, this imbalance still sets off alarms calling for chronic or long-term inflammation, and the immune system will respond accordingly. However, with no actual threat present, the immune system will start attacking things it normally wouldn't. This immune hypersensitivity can lead to a glut of problems ranging from simple allergies and weight gain to cancer, Alzheimer's disease, cardiovascular disease, diabetes, arthritis, asthma, prostate problems, and autoimmune diseases.

Many of these happen because as the immune system stays on high alert longer than it should, its agents begin to fatigue and make bad decisions, possibly leading to autoimmune disease or not destroying mutated cells, leading to cancer formation with more frequency. This can easily give way to cancer getting a foothold it won't easily relinquish.

Omega-3 fatty acids are clearly incredibly beneficial. Here are some omega-3 foods to include in your diet: flaxseeds and flaxseed oil, chia seeds, salba seeds, hemp seeds, fish (wild salmon, sardines, tongol tuna, herring, and cod), and fish oil. Obviously it's important to know which fats to eat and which ones to avoid when it comes to preventing those harmful prostaglandins I mentioned above.

What you eat is the single most important factor in quenching inflammation, and the healthiest way to eat is still sticking to what God has naturally provided for us on the earth. So, using an understanding of the Mediterranean diet that follows as a foundation, within that framework we will also look at pro-inflammatory and anti-inflammatory foods as well. If you are having problems with allergies, joint pains, muscle aches, or the like, by eating more anti-inflammatory foods than pro-inflammatory ones, you can tip your balance back in the right direction.

A GENTLE REMINDER

As we discussed earlier on, one way to check your degree of inflammation is to have a C-reactive protein (CRP) blood test. C-reactive protein is a promoter of inflammation and also a blood marker of systemic inflammation. Once you reach forty years of age, annual CRP testing is a great idea for checking the anti-inflammatory effectiveness of your diet. Men should aim for a CRP less than 1.0, while women should aim for a CRP less than 1.5.

The Mediterranean Diet: The Basic Building Block of Health

When I wrote a book about the Mediterranean diet, *What Would Jesus Eat?*, I learned that most Middle Easterners eat differently than the typical American. That sounds obvious, but what distinguishes the two isn't. I found that those who are used to a Mediterranean diet typically do not leave the dinner table stuffed as most Americans do. Generally they eat anything they want—but in moderation. They enjoy their food at a leisurely pace, socializing while eating. They have the uncanny ability to enjoy just a few bites of such foods as wine, dark chocolate, and chocolate ice cream. Unlike most Americans, who scarf down a dessert as if they were inhaling it, those eating the Mediterranean way generally savor just a few bites.

According to a 2003 study, "People who eat a Mediterranean-style diet rich in fruits, vegetables, whole grains, olive oil, and fish have at least a 25 percent reduced risk of dying from heart disease and cancer."[2] This is because the Mediterranean diet derives roughly 30 to 40 percent of its calories from healthy fats (coming from foods like olive oil, avocados, nuts, and fish) and about 40 to 50 percent from healthy carbohydrates like fruits, vegetables, beans, peas, lentils, and whole grains. Researchers also surmised that it was not any one component of this diet that makes it preventative, but it's the overall combination of foods, as well as avoiding foods that are potentially harmful, such as excessive calories from omega-6 oils, butter, sweets, and meats.

Combined with daily exercise, this is a powerful diet for living a longer and healthier life. Another study estimated that up to 25 percent of the incidence of colorectal cancer, about 15 percent of the incidence of breast cancer, and about 10 percent of the incidence of prostate cancer could be prevented if we shifted from a common Western diet to a traditional Mediterranean one.[3]

I believe the Mediterranean diet should be the foundation of your daily meal-planning here at the start, but you will need to make adjustments. Although breads and pastas are staples of the Mediterranean diet, I highly recommend that you avoid wheat and corn products at least until you have reached your desired waist measurement. You will also need to choose foods that do not create an inflammatory response in your body. But before we discuss what foods to avoid, let's first take a look at the primary foods in the Mediterranean diet:

- Extra-virgin olive oil—replaces most fats, oils, butter, and margarine. It is used in salads as well as for cooking. Extra-virgin olive oil strengthens the immune system. I recommend 4 tablespoons a day.
- Bread—consumed daily and prepared as whole-grain, dark, chewy, crusty loaves. I recommend waiting until you reach your desired weight or waist size to eat bread. At that point choose whole- and sprouted-grain breads such as Ezekiel 4:9 bread, but avoid white processed bread. (I do not recommend wheat or corn until you have achieved your desired waist measurement.)
- Thick, whole-grain pasta; brown or wild rice; couscous; bulgur; potatoes—often served with fresh vegetables and herbs, sautéed in olive oil, and occasionally served with small quantities of lean beef. Again, I recommend avoiding pasta and all wheat products to lose weight. Also limit the other starches to a tennis-ball serving, but no more than one of these starches per meal.
- Fruit—preferably raw, two to three pieces daily, but avoid bananas and dried fruit.

- Nuts—pecans, almonds, cashews, macadamia nuts, hazelnuts, and walnuts; preferably raw, and one handful a day.
- Beans—including pintos, great northern, navy, black, red, and kidney beans. Hummus, beans, and lentil soups are very popular (prepared with a small amount of extra-virgin olive oil). I recommend at least 1 to 4 cups of beans, peas, lentils, or hummus a day either as a soup or with the entree. (Beano helps prevent gas.)
- Vegetables—all types, including dark green variety, especially in salads, or eaten raw or steamed. Eat a large salad with extra-virgin olive oil and vinegar, and choose romaine, spinach, arugula, and the like, but do not choose iceberg lettuce. Iceberg lettuce is very low in fiber and nutritional content. Avoid the croutons.
- Small amounts of low-fat organic cheese and yogurt—cheese may be grated on soups or entrees. (The reduced-fat cheeses often taste better than the fat-free varieties. The best yogurt is Greek yogurt, fat free and organic without added fruit, but not frozen.) Also try grated feta or goat cheese in place of regular cheese.

CHOOSE OLIVE OIL WISELY

Do not buy extra-virgin olive oil packaged in a large plastic bottle. Olive oil is perishable, or it turns rancid. You should buy small amounts, packaged in dark glass bottles, and store it in a dark pantry at a cool temperature. Check expiration dates, and throw it away if it smells or tastes rancid.

In addition to eating the foods listed above, the following foods consumed a few times weekly make a good addition to the Mediterranean diet:

- Fish. The healthiest fish are cold-water varieties, such as cod, wild salmon, sardines, and tongol tuna. These are high in omega-3 fatty acids. Avoid farm-raised fish and high-mercury fish.
- Organic or free-range poultry. Poultry should be eaten two to three times weekly. Eat white breast meat with the skin removed.
- Organic or omega-3 eggs. These should be eaten only in small amounts (two to three per week). I recommend eating only one egg yolk with three egg whites and adding veggies to make an omelet cooked in extra-virgin olive oil once or twice a week.
- Organic or free-range lean red meat. Red meat should be eaten only rarely, on an average of once or twice a week. (I suggest consuming less than 12 ounces of red meat a week.) Use only lean cuts with the fat trimmed. Use in small amounts as an additive to spice up soup or pasta. (Note: The severe restriction of red meat in the Mediterranean diet is a radical departure from the American diet, but it is a major contributor to the low rates of cancer, heart disease, and stroke found in these countries.)

MERCURY LEVELS IN FISH

Although fish is generally a good protein choice, some fish contain high levels of mercury. The following list will help you determine which fish to eat more liberally and which to avoid.[4]

Fish with least amounts of mercury (enjoy these fish)

- Anchovies
- Sardines
- Catfish
- Shrimp
- Crab
- Sole
- Flounder
- Tilapia
- Haddock (Atlantic)
- Trout (freshwater)
- Herring
- Whitefish
- Salmon (fresh or canned)

Fish with moderate amounts of mercury (eat six servings or less per month)

- Bass (striped or black)
- Monkfish
- Halibut (Atlantic or Pacific)
- Snapper
- Tuna (canned, chunk light)
- Lobster
- Mahi-Mahi

Fish high in mercury (eat three servings or less per month)

- Bluefish
- Sea bass (Chilean)
- Grouper

- Tuna (canned albacore)
- Mackerel (Spanish and Gulf)
- Tuna (yellowfin)

Fish highest in mercury (avoid)

- Mackerel (king)
- Swordfish
- Marlin
- Tilefish
- Orange roughy
- Tuna (bigeye and ahi)
- Shark

Foods That Trigger Inflammation

Bad fats

Unfortunately the standard American diet swings the balance toward excessive amounts of bad prostaglandins. This can increase inflammation and constrict blood vessels, setting the stage for hypertension, heart disease, heart attack, stroke, weight gain, obesity, and diabetes.

While defenders of the dietary status quo poke fun at health advocates or ridicule them as the "food police," the truth is that there are dangers in the types of fats we consume. The main types that trigger inflammation are trans fats, hydrogenated fats, and partially hydrogenated fats. These are generally found in margarines, shortenings, hydrogenated oils, and most baked goods. They are especially prevalent in cake icing, many commercial peanut butters, chips, crackers, cookies, and any foods that list hydrogenated or partially hydrogenated oils on the label. Fried foods—especially those that are deep-fried (e.g., fried chicken, french fries, fried fish)—also increase inflammation.

You should also avoid excessive intake of saturated fats, which are found primarily in red meat, pork, processed meats, butter, whole milk, cheese, and poultry skins. All increase your chances of inflammation.

So do omega-6 fats, which are found in vegetable oils, such as safflower, corn, soy, sunflower, and cottonseed oils. Most salad dressings contain these toxic oils. Their labels will usually list "linoleic acid" or "polyunsaturated omega-6."

Corn-fed beef

Corn-fed beef significantly increases inflammation, which is why you should search for "organic" or "grass fed" designations on cuts of steak, hamburger, and other meats. What difference does it make? Grass-fed cattle have approximately six to eight times less fat than grain-fed cattle, as well as two to six times more omega-3 fats. These omega-3s decrease inflammation. This is because the grass the livestock eat typically contains omega-3 fats that are eventually stored in their flesh. Most livestock today are grain fed—usually corn. This increases the omega-6 oils, overall fat, and saturated fats. Both fats are inflammatory, which means that while you enjoy your hamburger or steak, you may be inflaming your body.

By the way, chickens are fed similar to the way livestock are fed. Feeding poultry a grain-based diet causes chickens, as well as their eggs, to be loaded with pro-inflammatory fats.

Sugars and refined carbohydrates

All sugars and refined carbohydrates can fan inflammation in the body. Refined carbohydrates include white bread, white rice, crackers, chips, refined sugary cereals, and potatoes. One study found that overweight women who ate these foods regularly had the highest levels of CRP.[5] Another study at Harvard University discovered that women who ate foods with the highest glycemic load (refined carbohydrates) experienced nearly twice as much inflammation as other women.[6] The more inflammation that exists in your body, the faster you will age and the more wrinkles you will develop. Try keeping that in mind the next time you reach for a soda, dessert, or white bread.

Foods rich in arachidonic acid

Both saturated fats and omega-6 fats can convert to arachidonic acid. Since this acid is a building block for bad prostaglandins, it is wise to limit consumption of this inflammatory fat. Foods rich in arachidonic acid include fatty cuts of red meat and pork, egg yolks, high-fat dairy products, shellfish, and organ meats.

The problem arises especially in men who consume a pound or two of steak, three to four eggs, a pint of ice cream, half a pound of cheese, a few tablespoons of butter, and a quart of whole milk daily. While periodically eating small portions (3 to 6 ounces) of lean, organic red meat is acceptable, eating mammoth-sized steaks or hamburger every day is a recipe for inflammatory disaster. When you eat large amounts of foods rich in arachidonic acid, your body increases its production of enzymes to break down the acid. This produces leukotriene B_4 and other inflammatory elements that can cause even more chronic inflammation.

Foods That Control Inflammation

Good fats

Just as bad fats are a source of inflammation, good fats are the best fire extinguishers. Omega-3 fats from cold-water fish, wild fish instead of farm-raised fish, or high-quality omega-3 supplements are the best anti-inflammatory oils. Unfortunately the standard American diet is low in omega-3 fats and high in the inflammatory omega-6 fats. The recommended ratio of omega-6 fats to omega-3 fats should be four to one. However, as I mentioned in the last chapter, most Americans consume these in a ratio closer to twenty to one!

FISHY TIP

When shopping for a great source of omega-3 fats to reduce inflammation, keep in mind that all salmon from Alaska is wild, whereas Atlantic salmon is typically farmed. Just because a grocery store or restaurant labels its salmon "wild" doesn't necessarily mean it is. Farmed fish makes up 90 percent of this country's salmon sales, so do your homework to make sure you can trust certain brands, supermarkets, or eating establishments.[7]

Another good fat that helps decrease inflammation is gamma linolenic acid, or GLA. Found in borage oil, black currant seed oil, and evening primrose oil, GLA is classified as an omega-6 oil but behaves more like an omega-3. Other good fats include the omega-9 family of fats; among them are olive oil, almonds, avocados, and macadamia nuts. In addition, raw nuts and seeds—such as walnuts, pecans, and flaxseeds—are good anti-inflammatory fats.

Increase fruits and vegetables

With the exception of potatoes and corn, almost all vegetables will help with inflammation. I recommend eating many different vegetables with a diversity of color—and choosing organic. Be aware that some vegetables classified as "nightshades" may trigger inflammation in some individuals, especially those with rheumatoid arthritis. Examples of nightshades are tomatoes, potatoes, peppers, and eggplants. If after eating nightshade vegetables you experience joint aches, swelling, or redness; rashes; or increased arthritis symptoms, you should probably limit or avoid nightshade vegetables. Sometimes the inflammation from eating these vegetables occurs within a day or two. For others, it may occur a few hours after consumption. If you suspect nightshades are causing inflammation, refer to www.worldhealth.net to find a physician experienced in diagnosing and treating food sensitivities.

Some fruits and vegetables are particularly helpful in calming inflammation. Onions, apples, red grapes, and red wine all contain quercetin, a powerful antioxidant that helps quench inflammation. Garlic, ginger, and rosemary sprigs have anti-inflammatory properties. So does curry powder, which contains curcumin, a highly anti-inflammatory spice. In addition, pineapple contains bromelain, an enzyme that decreases inflammation. The herb Boswellia also decreases inflammation. It's best to choose organic produce.

A sensible program like the one I recommend succeeds because it includes low-glycemic foods, including plenty of fruits and vegetables. A low-glycemic diet helps users practice portion control, limits bad fats, and encourages the consumption of healthy fats. Essentially, when you learn how to substitute good fats for inflammatory fats; replace high-glygemic, refined carbohydrates with low-glycemic, high-fiber ones; and eat lean, organic, free-range meats in place of high-fat, grain-fed varieties, you dramatically decrease inflammation. Limiting or avoiding sugar, juices, sodas, desserts, and sugary coffees can also help quench these fires.

The Anti-Inflammatory Diet: Taking the Mediterranean Diet to the Next Level

Using the Mediterranean diet as the foundation for your day-in, day-out meal planning, you can then balance your pro-inflammatory and anti-inflammatory foods as your body (and CRP tests, if you have taken them) indicates that you should. This will, of course, probably mean adding more anti-inflammatory foods and avoiding the pro-inflammatory ones for a time.

I have organized the following two lists of foods for you to consider adding or subtracting from your diet as your level of systemic inflammation demands.

TOP ANTI-INFLAMMATORY FOODS (ALWAYS CHOOSE ORGANIC WHEN POSSIBLE)	
Fruit	Raspberries, acerola (West Indian) cherries, guava, strawberries, cantaloupe, lemons/limes, rhubarb, kumquat, pink grapefruit, mulberries, blueberries, blackberries
Vegetables	Chili peppers, onions (including scallions and leeks), spinach, greens (including kale, collards, and turnip and mustard greens), sweet potatoes, carrots, garlic
Legumes	Lentils, green beans, peas
Egg products	Liquid eggs, egg whites (may use one organic or free-range egg yolk with three egg whites)
Dairy (use with caution)	Cottage cheese (low fat and nonfat), nonfat cream cheese, plain low-fat Greek yogurt or vanilla Greek yogurt (add fresh fruit if desired) (Limit dairy to 4–6 oz. every three to four days)
Fish	Herring, haddock, wild salmon (not farmed; Alaskan preferred), rainbow trout, sardines, anchovies (See Bible Cure Health Fact: Mercury Levels in Fish.)
Poultry	Goose, duck, free-range organic chicken and turkey (white meat preferred, skins removed) (3–6 oz. once or twice a day)
Meat	Eye of round (beef), flank steak, sirloin tip, skirt steak, pork tenderloin (free range preferred, extra lean or lean) (Limit to 3–6 oz. two times a week, 12 oz. max.)
Cereal	Steel-cut oatmeal, oat bran
Fats/oils	Safflower oil (high oleic), hazelnut oil, extra-virgin olive oil, avocado oil, almond oil, apricot kernel oil
Nuts/seeds	Brazil nuts, macadamia nuts, hazelnuts, pecans, almonds, hickory nuts, cashews (best raw)
Herbs/ spices	Garlic, onion, cayenne, ginger, turmeric, chili peppers, chili powder, curry powder, rosemary, ginger, boswellia
Sweeteners	Stevia, tagatose, coconut palm sugar
Beverages	Black, white, or green tea, club soda/seltzer, herbal tea, spring water
Starches	Sweet potatoes, new potatoes, millet bread, brown and wild rice, brown rice pasta, and legumes (see above for approved legumes)

INFLAMMATORY FOODS TO LIMIT OR AVOID	
Fruit	Mango, banana, dried apricots, dried apples, dried dates, canned fruits, raisins
Vegetables	White potatoes, french fries, potato chips
Legumes	Baked beans, fava beans (boiled), canned beans
Egg products	Duck eggs, goose eggs, hard-boiled eggs, egg yolks

INFLAMMATORY FOODS TO LIMIT OR AVOID	
Cheeses	Brick cheese, cheddar cheese, Colby cheese, cream cheese (normal and reduced fat)
Dairy	Fruited yogurt, ice cream, butter
Fish	Farm-raised fish and fish high in mercury (See Bible Cure Health Fact: Mercury Levels in Fish.)
Poultry	Turkey (dark meat), Cornish game hen, chicken giblets, chicken liver
Meat	Bacon, veal loin, veal kidney, beef lung, beef kidney, beef heart, beef brain, pork chitterlings, lamb rib chops, dark turkey meat with skin, turkey wing with skin, all processed meats
Breads	Hot dog/hamburger buns, English muffins, Kaiser rolls, bagels, french bread, Vienna bread, blueberry muffins, oat bran muffins
Cereal	Grape-Nuts, Crispix, Corn Chex, Just Right, Rice Chex, corn flakes, Rise Krispies, Raisin Bran, shredded wheat
Pasta/grain	White rice, lasagna noodles, macaroni elbows, regular pasta, all corn products except corn on the cob or frozen corn (non-GMO)
Fats/oils	Margarine, wheat germ oil, sunflower oil, poppy seed oil, grape seed oil, safflower oil, cottonseed oil, palm kernel oil, corn oil
Sweeteners	Honey, brown sugar, white sugar, corn syrup, powdered sugar
Crackers/ chips/ cookies	Corn chips, pretzels, graham crackers, saltines, vanilla wafers
Desserts	Sweetened condensed milk, angel food cake, chocolate and vanilla cake with frosting, chocolate chips, heavy whipping cream, ice cream, fruit leather snacks (Most all desserts are made with sugar.)
Candy	Hershey Kisses, jelly beans, Twix, Almond Joy, milk chocolate bars, Snickers
Beverages	Milk, Gatorade, pineapple juice, orange juice, cranberry juice, lemonade, sodas, sugar-laden soft drinks

These are not complete lists by any means—just some of the more likely "suspects" to watch out for and some of the more helpful helpers to work into your diet. As you read these now, some of them will jump out at you as things you like and need, but you don't have as much of them in your diet as you probably should. Others are the foods that it is time to change your habits about and say good-bye to. The thing to remember is that you have a choice about what you put in your mouth, and now that you have a little more knowledge about these foods, you can begin making healthier diet choices concerning them.

If you have no health problems or obesity, avoiding the inflammatory foods on the previous pages is a good general guideline; simply follow the Mediterranean diet I outlined earlier. Because your health is good, you have a little more freedom than someone who is struggling with his or her health or weight. You may eat some of the inflammatory foods listed, but I highly recommend you use moderation when consuming them.

If you have health problems or obesity, then in addition to understanding the anti-inflammatory and inflammatory food lists on the previous pages, I advise you to adhere to the following anti-inflammatory diet exactly as directed below and avoid all inflammatory foods. Once your health conditions clear up or you are able to maintain a healthy weight, you can ease up on the following guidelines. If you reintroduce wheat into your diet, choose whole-grain breads and sprouted breads such as Ezekiel 4:9 bread, and avoid white processed bread. But again use moderation whenever eating inflammatory foods.

DR. COLBERT'S ANTI-INFLAMMATORY DIET (ALWAYS CHOOSE ORGANIC WHEN POSSIBLE)	
Vegetables	• Steam, stir fry, or cook under low heat. • Best cooked with extra-virgin olive oil, macadamia nut oil, or coconut oil • Vegetable soups should be non-cream-based, low sodium (homemade is best); you may add some organic meat. • Juice your own vegetable juice; avoid store-bought juices, which are usually high in sodium.
Animal proteins (meat)	• 3 oz. once or twice a day for women; 3 to 6 oz. once or twice a day for men • Wild salmon, sardines, anchovies, tongol tuna, turkey (skin removed), free-range chicken (skin removed), eggs (omega-3 eggs as well) • When grilling, slice meat into thin slices; marinate in red wine, pomegranate juice, cherry juice, or curry sauce. Remove all char from meat. • Be cautious with egg yolks, keeping to a maximum of once or twice a week. You can combine one yolk with two to three egg whites. • Limit consumption of lean beef and red meat to one to two 3 to 6 oz. servings a week.
Fruits	• Berries, Granny Smith apples, lemon, or lime. If diabetic, choose only berries.
Nuts and seeds	• All raw nuts and seeds are acceptable, but just a handful once or twice a day.
Salads	• Use 1-calorie-per-spray salad spritzers; or create your own vinaigrette spritzer using a one to two ratio of extra-virgin olive oil to balsamic, apple cider, or red wine vinegar. So you would mix 1 to 2 Tbsp. extra-virgin olive oil with 2 to 4 Tbsp. vinegar. Once you attain a healthy weight and waistline, increase your olive oil to 4 Tbsp. a day in your salad dressing.
Dairy	• Low-fat dairy without sugar such as Greek yogurt and low-fat cottage cheese

DR. COLBERT'S ANTI-INFLAMMATORY DIET (ALWAYS CHOOSE ORGANIC WHEN POSSIBLE)	
Starches	• Sweet potatoes, new potatoes, brown/wild rice, millet bread, brown rice pasta • Two to four cups daily of beans, peas, legumes, lentils, or hummus • Use moderation when choosing starches, at most only one serving per meal, and make them the size of a tennis ball, not a basketball. • If diabetic, I recommend that you avoid starches.
Beverages	• Alkaline water or sparkling water; may add lemon or lime • Green, black, or white tea; may add lemon or lime • Coffee • Low-fat coconut milk or almond milk in place of cow's milk • No sugar; use stevia or other sugar substitutes such as Just Like Sugar, Sweet Balance, xylitol, chicory, or tagatose or coconut palm sugar in moderation. • No cream; use low-fat coconut milk.
Avoid	• Avoid all gluten (wheat, barley, rye, spelt); this includes all products made with these grains, including bread, pasta, crackers, bagels, pretzels, most cereals, etc. Go to www.celiacsociety.com for gluten-free foods. Also avoid corn products except for corn on the cob. Choose non-GMO.
Avoid	• Inflammatory animal proteins such as shellfish, pork, lamb, veal, and organ meats • Sugar • Fried foods • Processed foods • High-glycemic foods such as white rice, instant potatoes, etc.

Be sure to rotate your vegetables and meats every four days if you have food sensitivities. Do not eat the same food every day.

Additionally I highly recommend Monica Reinagel's *The Inflammation-Free Diet Plan*, where she presents her years of research to ascribe an inflammation-free (IF) rating to the foods we eat. This rating system takes into account more than twenty different factors that contribute to a food's relationship to inflammation. Positive ratings are anti-inflammatory, and foods with negative ratings promote inflammation. Up to one hundred on each scale is considered mildly one way or the other, over one hundred is moderate, and over five hundred is severe. Looking at her research and adding some of my own, I have organized the above two lists of foods for you to consider adding or subtracting from your diet as your level of systemic inflammation demands.

TOP TEN EXCUSES FOR NOT DIETING

1. "I just can't resist my favorite foods."
2. "My social life is just too crazy."
3. "I don't have time to lose weight or plan meals."
4. "My family and friends won't support me."
5. "I don't have anyone to hold me accountable."
6. "It's too confusing to find which diet works for me."
7. "I travel too much."
8. "Dieting is too restrictive."
9. "It's too expensive to diet."
10. "I'm just too impatient to diet."[8]

A Word About Portion Sizes

Any plan to lose weight will require you to limit your portions, but that doesn't mean you have to feel deprived. Barbara Rolls, PhD, introduced the concept of "volumetrics" as an answer to dieters who were sick of always feeling hunger. Her premise is simple: rather than eating tiny amounts of calorie-dense foods, eat lots of low-calorie foods that are naturally rich in water and fiber. Instead of bothering with counting calories or grams of fat, protein, or carbs, Rolls argues that dieters can eat more than they normally do and still lose weight—as long as they eat the right type of foods (ones that aren't calorie-dense).

Though I differ on many of her points, I believe Rolls is on to something by understanding that you can eat large portions of foods with little to no calories. Vegetables are a perfect example of this, which is why in this anti-inflammatory diet program you are essentially able to eat as many vegetables as you want with meals (minus the butter, of course).

In fact, there are a few simple volumetric tips you can use at every meal:

- Before every meal drink a tall glass of water with two or three capsules of PGX fiber. This usually prevents you from overeating.
- Enjoy a bowl of vegetable soup, minestrone soup, black bean soup, lentil soup, or any other broth-based, low-sodium, non-cream-based vegetable soup. A study done at Penn State concluded that eating a bowl of soup with an entree actually reduced the total consumed calories by 20 percent.[9] A cup of bean, pea, or lentil soup before your meal is very filling and will help you lose weight, but eat no more than four cups of beans, peas, and lentils per day.
- Precede your entree with a salad (any size). Make sure you use a salad spritzer with 1 calorie per spray. If you decide to eat your salad with extra-virgin olive oil and vinegar, be sure to limit your olive oil to 1 to 2 tablespoons and two or three times as much vinegar. You will use less if you use a salad spritzer. Avoid the croutons.
- Whether eating a salad or your entree, always remember to chew every bite twenty to thirty times; this not only helps your body digest and absorb the food's nutrients, but it also causes you

to eat slower and fill up faster. By prefilling your stomach with low-calorie foods, you are less likely to eat excess amounts of starches, meats, fats, and desserts.

DID YOU KNOW...?

Research has shown that people who successfully lose weight and keep it off eat breakfast every day. Other studies have gone a step further, proving that people who skip breakfast are prone to eating more food and snacks during the day.[10]

Unfortunately most Americans have their meals backward. We skimp on breakfast, eat a medium-size lunch, and then pig out come dinnertime. We should actually be doing the opposite. We should eat breakfast like a king (within thirty minutes of waking up), lunch like a prince, and dinner like a pauper.

Eat every three to three and a half hours to avoid hunger. Eating at the right times will leave you energized, mentally sharper, and more emotionally stable. Even your job performance will go up as a result.

Snacking Right

Ideally you should eat every three to three and a half hours to avoid hunger. Many people do not understand that a good snack can turn off your appetite and can stop the triggers from setting it off in the first place. And though it seems counterintuitive to some, snacking can help you burn more calories in the process. Researchers have determined that snacking on the right amount of healthy foods, in addition to eating three meals a day, boosts the metabolic rate more than if you only eat three meals each day.[11]

The best type of snack food is a mini-meal consisting of healthy protein; a high-fiber, low-glycemic carbohydrate or starch; and some good fat. When mixed together, this food fuel or fuel mixture is digested slowly, causing glucose to trickle into your bloodstream, which controls your hunger for hours.

Portion control is a key to wise snacking. Select half a serving of either a low-glycemic starch or one serving size of fruit. Then add 1 to 2 ounces of a protein and a third of a serving size of healthy fat. Typically this mini-meal should amount to just 100 to 150 calories for women and 150 to 250 calories for men.

Here are a few examples of well-rounded snacks.

Morning or afternoon snack

- 2 tablespoons of guacamole or avocado with raw carrots or celery
- 2 tablespoons of hummus with raw carrots or celery (4 inches in length)
- 10–15 baked lentil chips and 2 tablespoons of hummus, guacamole, or avocado (You can purchase the baked lentil chips at www.mediterraneansnackfoods.com.)
- 1 to 2 wedges of Laughing Cow Light cheese, 1 ounce of smoked salmon or tongol tuna (meat optional)
- Half a cup of nonfat cottage cheese, a piece of low-glycemic fruit (berries or Granny Smith apple), and 5 to 10 nuts
- A small salad with 1 to 2 ounces of sliced turkey and 2 tablespoons of avocado; use a salad spritzer or 1 tablespoon extra-virgin olive oil mixed with 2 to 3 tablespoons vinegar in a salad spritzer (meat optional)
- A bowl of broth-based vegetable, lentil, or bean soup with 1 to 2 ounces of boiled chicken
- A protein smoothie made from plant protein powder (1–2 scoops) mixed with 2 to 4 ounces of frozen berries and 8 ounces of low-fat coconut or

almond milk, or coconut kefir (option: dilute the coconut milk, almond milk, or kefir by reducing it to 4 ounces and combining with 4 ounces of filtered water or spring water)

Evening snacks

- Protein drink
- Lettuce wraps
- Salad with or without lean meat (may use a salad spritzer or one part extra-virgin olive oil mixed with two to three parts vinegar)
- Vegetable or bean or lentil soup with or without lean meat

Be sure to take two or three PGX fiber capsules with a 16-ounce glass of water with your snack. And remember you can add as many non-starchy vegetables as you want. To top it off, I recommend a cup of green or black tea, using natural stevia as a sweetener.

Keep plenty of healthy snack items at home, at work, and on the road. Always be prepared. And don't forget: it is important to get snacks that you truly enjoy. Otherwise you won't bother.

Tips for Eating Out

The National Restaurant Association estimates Americans spend 49 percent of their food budget at restaurants.[12] With America's fast-paced lifestyle, many parents feel they do not have time to prepare family meals, leading to an unhealthy reliance on fast-food restaurants. Meanwhile singles or couples without children at home have discovered that eating out regularly is easier and may be more economical. I don't recommend that you eat out all the time, but all of us will eat out from time to time—it is part of modern life.

The good news is that you can eat out and still enjoy a balanced, healthy meal. Most restaurants serve unhealthy food, so you can't eat just anything. In addition, portion sizes are often distorted. If you hope to control your weight, there are basic principles you must understand when deciding what dishes to order at restaurants.

- Choose sparkling water or unsweetened tea with a wedge of lemon or lime.
- Take two to four PGX fiber capsules with 16 ounces of unsweetened tea or water to help prevent overeating.
- Avoid the bread. If possible, ask that it not even be placed on the table.
- Choose an appetizer with vegetables and meats such as a shrimp cocktail. Avoid any that are deep-fried, high in starch and fats (i.e., quesadillas or corn bread), or bread based.
- Order your salad with the dressing on the side and with no croutons, cheese, or fattening side items. It's best to bring your own salad dressing spritzer or use olive oil and vinegar.
- Add a bowl of broth-based vegetable or bean or lentil soup to fill yourself up before the entrée.
- Choose entrées with meat, fish, or poultry that is baked, broiled, grilled, or stir-fried in a minimum amount of oil. Avoid anything deep fried or pan-fried. Meat portion sizes should be 3 ounces for women and 3 to 6 ounces for men. If the portion is larger, ask the server to put half in a to-go box.

- Limit sauces and gravies. If you must have them, ask that they be put on the side.
- Ask that vegetables be steamed without butter or oils (unless you prefer them raw).
- Choose sweet potato over white potato when possible. Because these are high-glycemic foods, keep portion to the size of a tennis ball.
- If you choose a dessert, share it and only take a few bites. Savor those bites.

One of the easiest ways to avoid sabotaging your weight-loss goals is planning. This will help you avoid unhealthy foods and overeating. Never go out to eat when you feel ravenous. I guarantee that you will eat too much of the wrong foods. Have a healthy snack such as a large Granny Smith apple or a pear before leaving the house. This will pre-fill your stomach and help prevent overeating.

In addition, plan what and where you will eat before leaving home. I also suggest patients plan an early dinner, usually between five and six o'clock, so they will finish early enough to burn off some calories before going to bed. You may also want to consider sharing an entrée with your spouse. Also be sure to slow down while eating, and chew every bite thoroughly, putting your fork down between bites. All these "little" things go a long way in controlling hunger and weight.

Fast-food restaurants

Choose a grilled chicken sandwich or a small hamburger. Throw away the top and bottom bun, and squeeze your burger between two napkins to remove excess grease. Cut the hamburger in half and then place both halves of the meat between two lettuce leafs. Avoid mayonnaise and ketchup; choose mustard, tomato, onions, and pickle. You can also order a small salad and ask for fat-free dressing (or use just a small portion of a regular packet). For a drink, order unsweetened iced tea or a bottle of water. Instead of french fries, order a baked potato when available, using only one pat of butter or 2 teaspoons of sour cream.

If you eat at a sub shop, choose turkey, lean roast beef, and chicken instead of bologna, pastrami, salami, corned beef, or other fatty selections. Choose a 6-inch sub, eating it with the smaller bottom of the bun and not the top portion. Use plenty of vegetables, and top with vinegar; avoid or go easy on the oil. It's best to further cut calories by ordering it in a lettuce or pita wrap.

MARATHON BURN

To burn off the 1,510 calories in a Quiznos large Chicken Carbonara, you'd have to expend the same calories it takes to bike across the state of Delaware (thirty miles).[13]

At fast-food chicken restaurants choose rotisserie or baked chicken instead of fried. Peel off the skin and pat the chicken dry with a napkin. Drain the liquid from the coleslaw, and do not eat the biscuit or potatoes.

Before diving into a slice of pizza, eat a large salad. Then have only one slice of pizza, sticking to thin or flatbread crust. Choose chunky tomatoes and other veggies as toppings. Avoid pepperoni and other highly processed meat toppings, and ask for half the cheese (the same way many ask for double cheese). Finally, use a napkin to remove excess oils from the cheese.

Italian restaurants

Start with a soup—minestrone, pasta fagioli, or broth-based tomato—and a large salad. Limit bread and olive oil, which has 120 calories per tablespoon. Good entrée options include grilled chicken, fish, shellfish, veal, and steak. Avoid fried or Parmesan dishes, such as chicken or veal Parmesan. Ask for your vegetables to be steamed, and avoid the pasta or have it cooked al dente, which causes it to have a lower glycemic index value. Don't overdo it on the pasta; the amount should be about the size of a tennis ball. Avoid fat-filled creamy sauces, cheese, and pesto sauce.

Mexican restaurants

Avoid the deep-fried tortilla chips, and choose tortilla soup without the chips or black bean soup as appetizers. Be wary of entrées smothered in melted cheese, which automatically increases the fat count. Choose fajitas with chicken, beef, or shrimp. Avoid the tortilla, and make your fajita with lettuce wraps. Add such ingredients as salsa, onions, lettuce, beans, and guacamole. Avoid cheese and sour cream if possible, since restaurants rarely serve nonfat varieties. As for beans, choose red or black but not refried, since they are high in fat. Avoid the rice. If a salad is available, enjoy a large one before your entrée.

ENSALADA

Just because a taco salad features the word *salad* doesn't mean it's healthy. With the massive fried tortilla shell, beef, cheese, sour cream, and additional items (plus the nutritionally useless iceberg lettuce), most taco salads add up to about 900 calories and 55 grams of fat.

Asian restaurants

These are usually good choices, provided your meat or seafood is baked, steamed, poached, or stir-fried. Steaming is usually the healthiest method. Instead of fried rice or fried noodles, choose brown rice. If permitted, substitute a serving of rice with vegetables. If that is not possible, don't eat more than a tennis-ball-sized serving of rice. Avoid sweet and sour, batter-fried, or twice-cooked food (which is high in fat and calories) and oily sauces (i.e., duck). For an appetizer you can choose wonton or egg drop soup instead of deep-fried egg rolls. Sushi is fine; some restaurants prepare it with brown rice.

Look for restaurants that do not use MSG or that will not use it on your dish. MSG has numerous potential reactions. The most common is stimulating your appetite, causing you to become hungry again in a couple hours. More importantly, MSG can lead to severe headaches, heart palpitations, and shortness of breath. (For more information on MSG, refer to my book *The Seven Pillars of Health*.)

Indian restaurants

Many Indian foods contain large portions of ghee (clarified butter) or oil, so it's best to find a restaurant willing to limit the amount they use on your dish. Tandoori-cooked (roasted) or grilled fish, chicken, beef, and shrimp are good choices. Avoid deep-fried foods and sauces, such as masala sauce and curry sauce, which are high in fat. If you must have them, get them in a small side dish. Also, it's best to avoid the breads—a major element of Indian food. If you have any, however, choose bread that is baked (*naan*) instead of the fried *chapatis* bread.

Family-style restaurants

Foods at these restaurants are typically high in fats; the main courses are often fried. The vegetables are usually loaded with gravy, butter, or oil. Good choices include baked or grilled chicken, turkey, or beef with steamed vegetables. Vegetable or bean or lentil soup and a salad (dressing on the side) also make good choices. Avoid the large dinner rolls, butter, and fried side dishes. Choose beans, such as lima, pinto, or string beans. If you must have gravy, get it on the side and eat it sparingly. Though raised on Southern cooking, I have learned I can enjoy the foods without all the gravies and fried options.

A Final Word

Eating healthily is not a diet but a lifestyle. So follow this lifestyle every day. There will be times that you will slip, especially on holidays, birthdays, anniversaries, weddings, and other special occasions. However, never give up. Simply get back on the program, and you will again start burning fat and building muscle.

If you reach a plateau or if you are unable to lose more weight, simply avoid high-glycemic carbohydrates, which include breads, pasta, potatoes, corn, rice, pretzels, bagels, crackers, cereals, popcorn, beans, bananas, and dried fruit. Choose low-glycemic vegetables and fruits. If after a month or two of doing this you are still unable to lose sufficient weight, you should choose low-glycemic vegetables and salads and avoid fruits for approximately a month until you break through the plateau. Then reintroduce low-glycemic fruits.

I am praying for God to give you the determination and willpower to follow through on this eating strategy. Not only will you reverse the stinging effects of inflammation in your body, but you will also lose weight—and keep it off! In doing so, you will take care of your body, God's temple, and live a full and abundant life to His glory. Eat right and live in divine health!

Action Steps

1. Which of the following healthy choices are you willing to make when you are eating out?
   - Plan ahead.
   - Eat a snack beforehand.
   - Take PGX fiber supplements beforehand.
   - Take half of the entrée to go.
   - Avoid dessert.
2. Keep a daily food diary, each day listing the date, your weight, and what you eat for breakfast, morning snack, lunch, afternoon snack, and dinner.

Chapter 9

GET YOUR EXERCISE GROOVE ON

God has made you the master of your body—it is not the master of you! Too many of us let our bodies tell us what to do. However, God created this incredible body to be your servant. The apostle Paul revealed his understanding of this truth when he said, "I discipline my body and bring it into subjection, lest, when I have preached to others, I myself should become disqualified" (1 Cor. 9:27).

God has given you the power of mastery over your body. If you've let inflammation take over your life, it's time to regain control. Proper diet and nutrition alone cannot reverse inflammation or reduce your weight sufficiently to control inflammation when it flares up. However, a healthy lifestyle that includes exercise will help you reach your goal of living pain free, inflammation free, and disease free.

Get Moving

There is no better way to complement a lifestyle change like that outlined in this book than with physical activity. It helps raise the metabolic rate during and after the activity. It enables you to develop more muscle, which raises the metabolic rate all day—even while you sleep. It decreases body fat and improves your ability to cope with stress by lowering the stress hormone cortisol.

DOG LOVERS?

Approximately 60 percent of dog owners do not walk their dogs, simply letting them out in the backyard.[1]

Such activity also raises serotonin levels, which helps reduce cravings for sweets and carbohydrates. It assists in burning off the dangerous belly fat that is a magnet for inflammation, and it improves your body's ability to handle sugar. Finally, regular physical activity can even help control your appetite by boosting serotonin levels, lowering cortisol, and decreasing insulin levels (which can also decrease your chances for insulin resistance). Simply put, regular activity is extremely important if you want to reverse inflammation while losing weight.

Before we continue, remember that it's important to see your personal physician before starting a rigorous exercise program. Even if you have health considerations, you may be surprised to learn there are ways for you to become more active. Cycling, swimming, dancing, hiking, and sports such as basketball, volleyball, soccer, and tennis are all considered aerobic. Washing the car by hand, working in your yard, and mowing the grass qualify too. An aerobic exercise is simply something that uses large muscle groups of the body and raises the heart rate to a range that will burn fat for fuel. This is why aerobic exercise is one of the best ways to lose body fat.

THE PERKS OF REGULAR ACTIVITY

In case you needed a reminder, here are some of the many benefits that regular activity promotes:

- It reduces chronic inflammation.
- It decreases the risk of heart disease, stroke, and the development of hypertension.
- It helps prevent type 2 diabetes.
- It helps prevent arthritis and aids in maintaining healthy joints.
- It helps prevent osteoporosis and aids in maintaining healthy bones.
- It helps protect you from developing certain types of cancer.
- It slows down the overall aging process.
- It improves your mood and reduces the symptoms of anxiety and depression.
- It increases energy and mental alertness.
- It improves digestion.
- It gives you more restful sleep.
- It helps prevent colds and flu.
- It alleviates pain.
- It promotes weight loss and decreases appetite.

Try brisk walking. Brisk walking is the simplest and most convenient way to exercise aerobically. Walk briskly enough so that you can't sing, yet slow enough so that you can talk. This is a simple way to ensure you are entering your target heart rate zone. Diabetic patients with foot ulcers or numbness in the feet may want to avoid walking and should try cycling, an elliptical machine, or pool activities while inspecting the feet before and after activity.

Aerobic exercise will make you feel better immediately by putting more oxygen into your body. It also tones the heart and blood vessels, increases circulation, boosts the metabolic rate, improves digestion and elimination, controls insulin production, stimulates the production of neurotransmitters in the brain, improves the appetite, and stimulates the lymphatic system, which aids in the removal of toxic material from the body.

NOT JUST NERVOUS

Fidgeting or getting up from your seat frequently can cause you to burn an additional 350 calories a day—which amounts to 36 pounds lost in a year![2]

Whatever activity you choose, the important thing is that you get moving regularly. Don't give yourself an excuse to justify a lack of activity. As you look for ways to increase your activity level, keep these tips in mind:

- Choose something that is fun and enjoyable. You will never stick to any activity program if you dread or hate it.
- Wear comfortable, well-fitting shoes and socks.
- If you are a type 1 diabetic, you will need to work with your doctor in order to adjust insulin doses while increasing your activity. Realize that exercising will lower your blood sugar; this can be potentially dangerous in a type 1 diabetic.
- The Centers for Disease Control and Prevention recommends brisk walking five days a week for thirty minutes. Start by walking only ten minutes a day and gradually increase your time to thirty minutes.

Recommended Level of Intensity

Every activity either requires or can be performed at different levels of intensity. Given that, it makes sense that every person hoping to lose weight has an ideal intensity at which he or she should work out. This is called your target heart rate zone, which generally ranges from 65 to 85 percent of your maximum heart rate.

To calculate the low end of this zone, start by subtracting your age from 220. This is your maximum heart rate. For example, for someone forty years old the formula is:

- 220 – 40 = 180 beats per minute

Multiply this number by 65 percent to find the low end of the target heart rate zone:

- 180 x 0.65 = 117 beats per minute

To figure out the high end of the zone, multiply maximum heart rate by 85 percent:

- 180 x 0.85 = 153 beats per minute

So, if you are forty, you should keep your heart rate between 117 and 153 beats per minute when exercising.

High-intensity aerobic exercise actually decreases insulin levels and increases levels of glucagon. By lowering insulin levels, you begin to release more stored body fat, and thus you burn fat, not carbohydrates. I recommend that you maintain a moderate pace as you exercise to keep your body burning fat as fuel.

When you exercise to the point that you are severely short of breath, you are no longer performing aerobically. Instead you have shifted to an anaerobic activity, which burns glycogen—stored sugar—as primary fuel instead of fat. I will explain the benefits of anaerobic activity a little later in this chapter. If you are just starting to exercise and aim to burn primarily fat, you need to work out at a moderate intensity of 65 to 85 percent of your maximum heart rate. This is the fat-burning range of your target heart rate zone.

When you start any activity program, I recommend you work out at around 65 percent of your maximum heart rate. As you become more aerobically conditioned, gradually increase the intensity to 70 percent of maximum heart rate. After a few more weeks increase to 75 percent, and so on. You may never be able to work out at 85 percent of maximum rate, especially if you are huffing and puffing. Be sure that as you increase the intensity of your workouts, you remain able to converse with another person.

DR. COLBERT APPROVED—SLEEP

Are you surprised to hear sleep is important? It is! Another way to stimulate release of growth hormone to build muscle is to get a good night's sleep. Growth hormone is secreted during stage three and stage four sleep, which occur during the first couple of hours after falling asleep.

Muscles and Metabolism

Have you thought that having a high metabolism was others' blessing but not yours? It can be. Your metabolic rate is dependent upon your muscle mass. The more muscle mass you have, the higher your metabolic rate. If your dieting efforts do not include exercise, you can begin to burn muscle mass to supply your body with amino acids and sabotage your weight-loss efforts by slowing down your metabolic rate. The body will then begin to burn fewer calories and less fat. The more muscle you carry, the higher the metabolic rate and the more stored body fat you will burn—even at rest. (And for a refresher on the way your metabolism works, revisit chapter 6.)

The Benefits of Anaerobic Exercise

Anaerobic exercise such as weight lifting, sprinting, and resistance training will help to increase lean muscle mass—thereby increasing your metabolic rate. If the workout is intense enough, growth hormone will be released from the pituitary gland. This leads to increased muscle growth and increased fat loss.

KEEPING TRACK

Researchers say that self-monitoring devices, such as a pedometer, heart rate monitor, or even a simple exercise journal can account for a 25 percent increase in successfully controlling your weight.[3]

For maximum results, however, the exercise must be very strenuous and done until muscle exhaustion occurs or until you simply cannot move any more. This stimulates the release of a powerful surge of growth hormone, which helps to repair and rebuild the muscles that have been broken down during the workout. As you gain more muscle mass, your metabolic rate rises.

A word of caution, however. If you weigh yourself, the scale may not show a dramatic weight loss since the muscle mass that you are adding actually weighs more than the fat it is replacing.

I encourage my patients not to begin resistance training until they are in the routine of walking approximately thirty minutes five days a week. If you are just beginning a weight-lifting program, I recommend that you consult a certified personal trainer who will develop a well-rounded weight-lifting program for you.

As you exercise, be sure to maintain proper form and lift the weights slowly to avoid injury. You should typically perform ten to twelve repetitions per set. When starting resistance training, I recommend only performing one set per activity to reduce soreness. As you become better conditioned over time, you can increase to two or three sets per activity.

WHEN ACTIVITY ITCHES

For most people, food allergy symptoms arrive shortly (if not immediately) after consuming a particular food with allergens. However, for a small segment of the population, such a reaction is conditional on physical activity. Those who have a physical-activity-induced food allergy only detect it if they eat a certain food or foods and then work out. As their body temperature increases, symptoms such as itching, lightheadedness, hives, asthma, or anaphylaxis can appear. The remedy is as easy as not eating for at least two hours before an activity session.

Increased sugar and increased starch will inhibit growth hormone release and is counterproductive. Therefore, prior to a workout, avoid snacks that are high in sugar or carbohydrates since you will not have the advantage of this powerful hormone for fat loss and muscle gain.

High-intensity interval training (HIIT) can also be an effective anaerobic workout. HIIT is simply alternating between brief, hard bursts of exercise and short stretches of lower-intensity exercise or rest, usually for a period of less than twenty minutes. Various studies in recent years have proven this to be an effective way to improve not only overall cardiovascular health but also your ability to burn fat faster. One study at the University of Guelph in Ontario, Canada, found that following an interval training session with an hour of moderate cycling increased the amount of fat burned by 36 percent.[4]

I personally do HIIT three times a week. I warm up on the elliptical machine for five to ten minutes. I then do sixty seconds of high-intensity training with high resistance and as fast as I can. I then decrease the resistance and speed to a lower setting for one minute. I continue this pattern for twenty minutes or more.

High-intensity anaerobic workouts obviously have proven value. However, I suggest that you hold off on HIIT, regardless of your exercise past, until you've consistently done some moderate-intensity activity for several months. I'd rather see you be able to sustain your momentum for the long haul rather than have you burn out, not because of eating the wrong things, but simply because you wanted to sprint to the finish line faster.

Be sure to have a physical exam with an EKG and/or a stress test before starting HIIT.

How Much Exercise Is Enough?

The Centers for Disease Control and Prevention and the National Institutes of Health recommend that adults need two types of physical activity each week—aerobic and muscle-strengthening. For aerobic activity they recommend two hours and thirty minutes of moderate intensity aerobic activity (brisk walking, water aerobics, riding a bike on level ground, playing doubles tennis, pushing a lawn mower, etc.) every week, or one hour and fifteen minutes of vigorous exercise (jogging, swimming laps, riding a bike fast or on hills/inclines, playing singles tennis, playing basketball, etc.) every week. For muscle-strengthening exercise, which I call resistance exercise, they recommend two or more days a week, working all major muscle groups (legs, hips, back, abdomen, chest, shoulders, and arms).[5]

I recommend breaking up the aerobic activity as follows. If you can only do moderate intensity activities, try brisk walking for thirty minutes a day, five days a week. If you can handle more vigorous activity, jog for twenty-five minutes a day, three days a week. Or you can break it down even further: try going for a ten-minute walk, three times a day, five days a week.

DR. COLBERT APPROVED—MONITOR YOURSELF

I believe in monitoring yourself on progress. An excellent way to monitor the steps you walk during the day is by using a pedometer. Typically a person walks three thousand to five thousand steps a day. To stay fit, set a goal of ten thousand steps, or approximately five miles. To lose weight, aim for between twelve thousand and fifteen thousand steps per day.

Before engaging in any activity, make sure that you have either eaten a meal two or three hours prior or have had a healthy snack about thirty to sixty minutes beforehand. It is never good to work out when hungry; you may end up burning muscle protein as energy—which is very expensive fuel. Remember, losing muscle lowers your metabolic rate.

If you lose weight steadily and then seem to hit a plateau, exercise will help. By increasing the frequency and duration of exercise, you can break through that plateau and continue losing weight. Try to increase your exercise time gradually from thirty minutes to forty-five minutes. Those stubborn last few pounds will soon begin to melt away.

Your body is a wonderful gift. With God's help you can get into shape, feel better, and look fabulous. Determine right now to put these exercise tips into practice and, most importantly, to stay with it. Remember, everyone falls down, but it takes an individual with courage to get back up again. You will have your ups and downs—we all do. But hang in there. Stay with it. Before long you'll be feeling the wonderful effects of living a life free of inflammation!

Action Steps

1. Which of the following lifestyle changes are you willing to make to achieve weight loss:

    - Exercise regularly.
    - Get enough sleep.
    - Begin a strengthening program.
    - Secure an accountability or exercise partner.

2. What exercise program are you committed to starting right away?

Chapter 10

SUPPORT IT WITH SUPPLEMENTS

Your body is also the most incredible creation in the entire universe. All the money in the world could not replace it. It's God's awesome gift and a suitable place to house His own Spirit. Since your body was created as the temple of God's Spirit, it's important to understand that you and I are merely stewards of this gift God has given us.

If you went out today and purchased a Mercedes-Benz or a Porsche, no doubt you would polish it and fill it with the best gas and the best oil—treating it with the respect that such a fine machine deserves. You can honor God in your body as well by treating it with the respect and care that befits such a wonderful gift.

By giving your body the nutrients, vitamins, and minerals it needs to function at peak performance, you will bring honor to God by properly caring for your body—the temple He created to house His own Spirit on this earth.

What Is Your Body Trying to Tell You?

Your incredible body is so sophisticated that it is programmed to signal you that it needs a nutrient or a vitamin you haven't supplied. These signals come in the form of cravings. Have you ever just had to have a glass of orange juice? Your body was probably telling your brain that it needed more vitamin C.

Cravings can come following a meal when the body realizes

that, although it's been fed, it still hasn't received enough of the nutrients it expected. Too often, instead of discerning the craving properly, we simply fuel our bodies with even more non-nutritious food. Therefore the cravings return, and we respond once again with more junk food. The cycle becomes vicious, we get fatter, and our bodies suffer for lack of real nutrition.

If you experience such cravings, it's likely your body is actually slightly malnourished. Vitamins, minerals, and supplements are vital in today's world for the proper fueling of our bodies. You see, most old-time farmers know that in order for soil to supply the food it produces with a rich supply of vitamins and minerals, it must rest or lie fallow. In other words, it must remain unused every few years. In today's world of high-tech agriculture, this no longer occurs. Therefore our food supplies are actually depleted of the vitamins, minerals, and nutrients our bodies need to maintain good health. So we give our bodies more and more food, but they still lack vitamins and nutrients. That's where supplementation can bridge the gap.

WILLING TO PAY

Sales of weight-loss drugs in the United States have surpassed the $1 billion mark, crossing that threshold in the fall of 2010.[1]

Natural Supplements for You

Let's explore some of these natural substances that can promote health and vitality as you defeat obesity in your life. Since there are many causes of obesity, I recommend safe nutritional supplements that work through different mechanisms, such as thermogenic agents, natural appetite suppressants that increase satiety, supplements that increase insulin sensitivity, and energy products. We will also look at some of the supplements you should avoid as you take the necessary steps to reach your ideal weight in reversing inflammation.

Vitamins and minerals

A good multivitamin and multimineral. It's important to be sure that you get a good supply of all the various vitamins your body needs, especially if it is depleted. Most multivitamins contain only twelve vitamins in their inactive form. You may want to choose a multivitamin you can take two to three times a day.

To prevent our adrenal glands from becoming exhausted, we need to supplement our diets daily with a comprehensive multivitamin and mineral formula with adequate amounts of B-complex vitamins. Divine Health Active Multivitamin has the active form of the vitamins, chelated minerals, and antioxidants in a balanced comprehensive formula.

Choosing a mineral supplement is a little more difficult than choosing a vitamin supplement—and sometimes more costly. Find a mineral supplement that is chelated rather than one that contains mineral salts. Chelation is a process of wrapping a mineral with an organic molecule such as an amino acid that increases absorption dramatically. (See appendix.)

Green Supreme Food. This supplement contains fifteen organic fruits, veggies, and superfoods, as well as probiotics, fiber, antioxidants, and phytonutrients. It helps energize, detoxify, and create an alkaline environment in the tissue, helping you lose weight.

Thermogenic (fat-burning) agents

The term *thermogenic* describes the body's natural means of raising its temperature to burn off more calories. More specifically, thermogenesis is the process of triggering the body to burn white body fat, which is the kind of fat we often accumulate as we age. Thermogenic agents, then, are fat burners that help to increase the rate of white-body-fat breakdown. Fortunately, most unsafe thermogenic agents have been pulled off the market.

Green tea. Green tea and green tea extract are good weight-loss supplements. Green tea has been used for thousands of years in Asia as both a tea and an herbal medicine. It has two key ingredients: a catechin called epigallocatechin gallate (EGCG) and caffeine. Both lead to the release of more epinephrine, which then increases the metabolic rate. Ultimately green tea promotes fat oxidation, which is fat burning. It also increases the rate at which you burn calories over a twenty-four-hour period.

An effective daily dose of EGCG is 90 mg or more, which can be consumed by drinking three or four cups of green tea a day. Do not add sugar, honey, or artificial sweeteners to it, though you may use the natural sweetener stevia. In addition to drinking green tea, I recommend 100 mg of green tea supplement three times a day. (See appendix.)

GREEN IS GOOD

A study found that after three months of taking green tea extract, overall body weight declined 4.6 percent while waist circumference decreased by nearly 4.5 percent.[2]

Green coffee bean extract. A placebo-controlled study reported in January 2012 that green coffee bean extract produced weight loss in 100 percent of overweight participants. For twenty-two weeks participants were given 350 mg of green coffee bean extract twice a day. They did not change their diets, averaging 2,400 calories per day, but they did burn 400 calories a day through exercise. The average weight loss was 17.6 pounds, with some subjects losing 22.7 pounds, and there were no side effects.[3]

The key phytonutrient in green coffee bean extract is chlorogenic acid, which has the ability to decrease the uptake of glucose, fats, and carbohydrates from the intestines and thus decrease the absorption of calories. It also has positive effects on how your body processes glucose and fats, and it helps to lower blood sugar and insulin levels. Drinking coffee doesn't give you the same effects. Because of roasting, most of the chlorogenic acid in coffee is destroyed. By comparison, the extract is much better. Green coffee bean extract should contain 45 percent or more of chlorogenic acid. In addition to—or in place of—drinking coffee, I recommend taking 400 mg of green coffee bean extract thirty minutes before each meal. (See appendix.)

Meratrim. Meratrim is a blend of two plant extracts that has been shown to significantly reduce body weight, BMI, and waist measurement within eight weeks when used with a diet and exercise plan. The studies show that 400 mg of Meratrim twice a day, thirty minutes before breakfast and thirty minutes before dinner, achieved these results by interfering with the accumulation of fat while simultaneously increasing fat burning.[4] (See appendix.)

Thyroid support

All obese patients should be screened for hypothyroidism, using tests such as the blood tests TSH, free T3, free T4, and thyroid peroxidase antibodies, to rule out Hashimoto's thyroiditis, the most common cause of low thyroid. If a patient has low body temperature (less than 98 degrees), they most likely have a sluggish metabolism and may have sluggish thyroid function. It's especially important to optimize the free T3 blood level to improve the metabolic rate. The normal range of T3, according to the lab I use, is 2.1 to 4.4. I try to optimize the T3 level to a range of 3.0 to 4.2 by using both levothyroxine (T4) and liothyronine (T3). I can sometimes optimize the T3 levels with natural supplements including Metabolic Advantage or iodine supplements. I also commonly perform a lab test to see if a patient is low in iodine before starting iodine supplements. According to the American Thyroid Association, 40 percent of the world's population is at risk for iodine deficiency.[5]

Appetite suppressants

These supplements generally act on the central nervous system to decrease appetite or create a sensation of fullness. Although some medications in this category include risk-prone phenylpropanolamine (found in such products as Dexatrim), I have found a few safe, natural supplements that are extremely effective appetite suppressants.

L-tryptophan and 5-HTP. These are amino acids that help the body to manufacture serotonin. Serotonin assists in controlling carbohydrate and sugar cravings. L-tryptophan and 5-HTP also function like natural antidepressants. If you are taking migraine medications called triptans or SSRIs (selective serotonin reuptake inhibitors), you should talk with your physician before taking either supplement. The typical dose of L-tryptophan is 500 to 2,000 mg at bedtime. For 5-HTP it is typically 50 to 100 mg one to three times a day or 100 to 300 mg at bedtime. Serotonin Max is an excellent supplement that helps boost serotonin levels naturally. (See appendix.)

L-tyrosine, N-acetyl L-tyrosine, and L-phenylalanine. These are naturally occurring amino acids found in numerous protein foods, including cottage cheese, turkey, and chicken. They help to raise norepinephrine and dopamine levels in the brain, which then helps decrease appetite and cravings and improves your mood. Doses of L-tyrosine, N-acetyl L-tyrosine, and L-phenylalanine may range from 500 to 2,000 mg a day (sometimes higher), but they should be taken on an empty stomach. I prefer N-acetyl L-tyrosine for most of my patients since the body absorbs it better than L-tyrosine or L-phenylalanine. I typically start patients on 500 to 1,000 mg of N-acetyl L-tyrosine, taken thirty minutes before breakfast and thirty minutes before lunch. I do not recommend taking any of these supplements in late afternoon because they may interfere with sleep. (See appendix.)

Supplements to increase satiety

Fiber supplements and foods high in fiber increase feelings of fullness by using several different mechanisms. Fiber slows the passage of food through the digestive tract, decreases the absorption of sugars and starches into the stomach, and expands and fills up the stomach—turning down the appetite. Although the American Heart Association and the National Cancer Institute recommend 30 grams or more of fiber each day, the average American only consumes between 12 and 17 grams.[6]

When it comes to losing weight and managing blood sugar levels, a little fiber goes a long way. One study found that consuming an extra 14 grams of soluble fiber each day for only two days was associated with a 10 percent decrease in caloric intake.[7] Soluble fiber supplements significantly increase post-meal satisfaction and should be taken before each meal to assist in weight loss. Soluble fiber lowers the blood sugar, slowing down digestion and the absorption of sugars and carbohydrates. This allows for a more gradual rise in blood sugar, which lowers the glycemic index of the foods you eat. This helps to improve the blood sugar levels.

The fiber that I prefer for weight-loss patients is PGX. I start with one capsule, taken with 8 to 16 ounces of water before each meal and snack, and then gradually increase the dose to two to four capsules until patients can control their appetite. Always take PGX with evening meals and snacks.

In addition to PGX, another great fiber for weight loss is glucomannan, made from the Asian root konjac. Glucomannan is five times more effective in lowering cholesterol when compared to other fibers such as psyllium, oat fiber, or guar gum. Because it expands to ten times its original size when placed in water, it is a great supplement to take before a meal to reduce your appetite as it expands in your stomach, but you should take it with 16 ounces of water or unsweetened black or green tea. (See appendix.)

WHAT'S THE POINT IF A PILL CAN DO IT?

Marketing researchers have found that the more proven a drug is to be effective at shedding pounds, the more lax the efforts of the user at continuing to eat well and exercise. Those who take prescription or over-the-counter diet pills are more likely to engage in eating junk food and living a sedentary lifestyle.[8]

Supplements to increase energy production

L-carnitine is an amino acid that helps our bodies turn food into energy by shuttling fatty acids into the mitochondria, which act as our cells' energy factories by burning fatty acids for energy. Humans synthesize very little carnitine, so we may need to supplement from outside sources. This applies especially to obese and older individuals, who typically have lower levels of carnitine than the average-weight segment of the population. As you might expect, individuals with insufficient carnitine have a greater difficulty burning fat for energy.

Milk, meat such as mutton and lamb, fish, and cheese are good sources of L-carnitine. I recommend taking a combination of L-carnitine and acetyl-L-carnitine, lipoic acid, PQQ (pyrroloquinoline quinone), and a glutathione-boosting supplement. The best time to take these supplements is in the morning and early afternoon (before 3:00 p.m.) on an empty stomach. If you take them any later, these supplements can impair your sleep. Green tea supplements and N-acetyl L-tyrosine also help to increase your energy.

Other common supplements to assist with weight loss

Irvingia. Irvingia is a fruit-bearing plant grown in the jungles of Cameroon in Africa. Irvingia gabonensis helps to resensitize your cells to insulin. It appears to be able to reverse leptin resistance by lowering levels of C-reactive protein (CRP), an inflammatory mediator. Leptin is a hormone that tells your brain you've eaten enough and that it is time to stop. It also enhances your body's ability to use fat as an energy source. You also need zinc, 12 to 15 mg a day, which is present in most comprehensive multivitamins, in order for leptin to function optimally.

Because of Americans' sedentary lifestyles and highly processed, high-glycemic food choices, many overweight and obese patients have acquired resistance to leptin. As a result, this hormone no longer works properly in their bodies. Similar to insulin resistance, leptin resistance is a chronic inflammatory condition that contributes to weight gain. It is critically important to follow the anti-inflammatory dietary program I have outlined in this book. Simply decreasing inflammatory foods enables most to start losing belly fat and also allows leptin to function optimally. The generally recommended dose is 150 mg of standardized Irvingia extract, twice a day, thirty minutes before lunch and dinner.

7-keto-DHEA. Derived from the hormone dehydroepiandrosterone (DHEA), 7-keto-DHEA is taken to help rev a person's metabolism to aid in weight loss. Unlike its "parent hormone" DHEA, which is produced by glands near the kidneys, 7-keto-DHEA does not affect sex hormone levels in the body.[9] The supplement is also used to improve lean body mass, build muscle, boost the immune system, enhance memory, and slow aging, though there is limited scientific evidence to support all of those benefits.[10] However, 7-keto-DHEA has been shown to increase the resting metabolic rate in those who were already dieting and engaging in regular exercise. An eight-week study found that those who took 100 mg of 7-keto-DHEA twice a day lost about six pounds, while those who received a placebo lost a little over two pounds.[11] The supplement was not found to have any adverse side effects after a series of toxicological evaluations. A safety study published in *Clinical Investigative Medicine* indicated that 7-keto-DHEA was safe for human consumption in doses of 200 mg per day for up to four weeks. The safety of internal use beyond four weeks is not known.[12]

The hoodia controversy. Hoodia is a South African plant similar to a cactus that may help suppress the appetite. Initially used by tribal leaders to enable them to go on long journeys without getting hungry, various sources cite thousands of years' worth of Bushman history to verify its effectiveness. Although these tribal hunters obviously have not conducted scientific studies to prove hoodia is an effective appetite suppressant, one 2001 clinical study by a company called Phytopharm found individuals who consumed the plant ate 1,000 fewer calories a day than those who didn't take hoodia.[13] One of the company's researchers, Richard Dixey, MD, explained that hoodia contains a molecule that is ten thousand times more active than glucose.[14]

However, there is a catch. When news of this supposed miracle supplement hit the headlines, dozens (if not hundreds) of companies started marketing hoodia—without having any actual hoodia in their products. The result was that more hoodia was "produced" in a single year than in all of African history—highly unlikely, to say the least. Even today it is possible that much of what is sold in the United States either contains ineffective hoodia variations or no hoodia. So be wary of falling for marketing schemes with this substance.

No Magic Bullet

There is no magic weight-loss pill. Scientists have been searching for "The Pill to End All Diets" for years, and no magic bullet has been found. There have been several attempts, including the popular fen-phen back in the nineties. While individuals lost weight, after only a few years a small percentage of users died of a rare disease called primary pulmonary hypertension. This affected several patients out of one hundred thousand; about half of them eventually required a heart-lung transplant to survive. The drug was eventually pulled, and several years later another "miracle cure" seemed to emerge. Combining ephedra with caffeine seemed to be a powerful formula for turning down the appetite and burning fat. But in time the safety of ephedra was also called into question. It has been linked with severe side effects, including arrhythmias, heart attack, stroke, hypertension, psychosis, seizure, and even death.

Due to safety concerns, in 2004 the Food and Drug Administration banned ephedra products in the United States. Although a federal court later upheld the ban, companies wiggle around it by selling extracts that contain little or no ephedrine. And some related herbs, such as bitter orange (citrus aurantium) and country mallow, remain on the market. Like ephedra, bitter orange supplements have been linked to stroke, cardiac arrest, angina, heart attack, ventricular arrhythmias, and death. These products are potentially lethal. I do not recommend them unless taken under the direction and close monitoring of a knowledgeable physician.

ALLI AND HYDROXYCUT SIDE EFFECTS

Alli, one of the most common over-the-counter diet pills, may cause bowel changes in its users. These changes, which result from undigested fat going through the digestive system, may include gas with an oily discharge, loose stools or diarrhea, more frequent and urgent bowel movements, and hard-to-control bowel movements.

Hydroxycut products were recalled in May 2009 after reports of deadly liver failure and disease in individuals who took the products to lose weight. According to the *World Journal of Gastroenterology*, an ingredient in Hydroxycut from a fruit called Garcinia cambogia caused the liver disease and failure.[15]

Among other herbs of concern is aristolochia, which is found in some Chinese herbal weight-loss supplements and may not even be listed as an ingredient. Aristolochia is a known kidney toxin and carcinogen in humans. There are also products containing usnea (usnic acid), a lichen for weight loss that can cause severe liver toxicity. In addition, some Brazilian diet pills have been found to be contaminated with amphetamines and other prescription drugs.[16]

A weight-loss supplement is a nutritional product or herb intended to assist your healthy eating and activity plan with the ultimate goal of losing weight. A supplement comes alongside; it does not replace. Do not be deceived by crafty marketing that promises otherwise. Weight-loss and dietary supplements are not subject to the same standards as prescription drugs or medications sold over the counter. They can be marketed with only limited proof of safety or effectiveness.

A Lifestyle Choice

While some questionable products are on the market, there are a variety of safe, effective over-the-counter dietary supplements for weight loss. Some people may find that incorporating a combination of these into their eating and activity plan works even better. Others may not need to take any supplements.

Most of my overweight and obese patients have found that taking a combination of green tea extract, green coffee bean extract, and Irvingia (see appendix) along with certain amino acids (such as Serotonin Max and N-acetyl L-tyrosine) and PGX fiber supplements before each meal and snack (especially in the evening) helped them shed pounds and controlled their appetites. (See appendix.)

If you continue experiencing problems controlling your appetite or struggle with food cravings, decreased energy, or insulin resistance, you will likely require one or more of the supplements I just reviewed. The same goes if you do not feel full or satisfied after a meal or if you have low hormone levels.

However, I remind you that supplements are just that—supplements, not magic pills. The truth is that there is no shortcut to losing weight and keeping it off. A new lifestyle that includes good nutrition, exercise, supplementation, and constant diligence is the best way to reverse inflammation and lose weight associated with it. The vitamins and supplements I have suggested can help you, but only you can decide to begin an entirely new lifestyle filled with health, vitality, and God's very best! Make that determination at this very moment. Make that commitment for your very life.

Action Steps

1. Which of the following steps are you willing to take:
   - Take a multivitamin.
   - Drink green tea or take green tea extract.
   - Use fiber.
   - Take green coffee bean extract.
2. What are the diligent ways you have already begun living in divine health?
3. What lifestyle changes are still left for you to do?

A PERSONAL NOTE FROM DON COLBERT

God desires to heal you of disease. His Word is full of promises that confirm His love for you and His desire to give you His abundant life. His desire includes more than physical health for you; He wants to make you whole in your mind and spirit as well as through a personal relationship with His Son, Jesus Christ.

If you haven't met my best friend, Jesus, I would like to take this opportunity to introduce Him to you. It is very simple. If you are ready to let Him come into your life and become your best friend, all you need to do is sincerely pray this prayer:

> *Lord Jesus, I want to know You as my Savior and Lord. I believe You are the Son of God and that You died for my sins. I also believe You were raised from the dead and now sit at the right hand of the Father praying for me. I ask You to forgive me for my sins and change my heart so that I can be Your child and live with You eternally. Thank You for Your peace. Help me to walk with You so that I can begin to know You as my best friend and my Lord. Amen.*

If you have prayed this prayer, you have just made the most important decision of your life. I rejoice with you in your decision and your new relationship with Jesus. Please contact my publisher at pray4me@charismamedia.com so that we can send you some materials that will help you become established in your relationship with the Lord. We look forward to hearing from you.

Appendix

RESOURCE GUIDE FOR REVERSING INFLAMMATION

Most of the products mentioned throughout this book are offered through Dr. Colbert's Divine Health Wellness Center or are available at your local health food store.

Divine Health Nutritional Products

1908 Booth Circle
Longwood, FL 32750
Phone: (407) 331-7007
Website: www.drcolbert.com
E-mail: info@drcolbert.com

Maintenance nutritional supplements

- Divine Health Multivitamin
- Divine Health Living Multivitamin
- Max N-Fuse

Heart health

- Living CoQ_{10}
- Plant bark extract and grape seed extract—OPCs
- LipiControl

Diabetic support

- PGX Fiber

- Cinnulin PF (cinnamon extract)
- Divine Health Fiber
- Divine Health Nutrients for Glucose Regulation
- Divine Health Vitamin D_3, 2,000 IU
- Chromium, 200 mcg
- Alpha lipoic acid (ALA Max, 600 mg capsule)
- Diaxinol (alpha lipoic acid, cinnulin, chromium, biotin, gymnema, and vanadyl sulfate)—Dr. Colbert's favorite supplement for diabetics

Omega oils

- Divine Health Living Omega
- Ultra Krill

Recommended natural sweeteners

- Stevia
- Just Like Sugar

Protein powders

- Divine Health Undenatured Whey Protein
- Plant protein

Supplements for weight loss

- Irvingia
- PGX Fiber
- Glucomannan
- Living Green Tea with EGCG
- Living Green Coffee Bean
- Meratrim (Metabolic Lean)

Supplements for thyroid support

- Metabolic Advantage

To curb food cravings

- Serotonin Max
- Advanced fat loss drops
- N-acetyl L-tyrosine
- L-tyrosine
- L-phenylalanine
- L-tryptophan
- 5-HTP

Other supplements

- DIM
- Indole-3-carbinol
- Beta TCP
- Divine Health Probiotic
- Divine Health Fiber Formula
- Serotonin Max
- Beta TCP
- L-carnitine with lipoic acid and PQQ (Mitochondria Basics with PQQ)

Glutathione boosters

- Max GXL
- Max One
- Cellgevity—Dr. Colbert's favorite glutathione booster

Snack bars

- Nutiva Hemp Chocolate Bars

Other Resources

- Sage Medical Lab, ALCAT, and NAET for delayed food allergy/sensitivity testing. Visit their websites at www.sagemedlab.com, www.alcat.com, and www.naet.com.
- For knowledgeable doctors in bioidentical hormone replacement (make sure they are board certified in anti-aging): www.worldhealth.net
- Chelation therapy—call 1-800-LEADOUT
- Grissini breadsticks, which are available at most grocery stores
- hCG sublingual tablets, which must be prescribed by a physician. (Physicians, call Pharmacy Specialist at (407) 260-7002.)
- Certified personal trainer. Lee Viersen is my personal trainer, and he can be reached through his website at www.LeeViersen.com or by phone at (407) 435-7059.

NOTES

Introduction
What Is Inflammation?

1. Wikipedia.org, s.v. "List of Wildfires: North America," http://en.wikipedia.org/wiki/List_of_wildfires#North_America (accessed October 29, 2014).

Chapter 1
Heart Disease

1. WebMD.com, "How the Heart Works," February 24, 2014, http://www.webmd.com/heart-disease/guide/how-heart-works (accessed October 29, 2014).
2. Michigan State University, Department of Physics and Astronomy, "How Long Does It Take Your Heart to Circulate the Total Amount of Blood in Your Body?", http://www.pa.msu.edu/sciencet/ask_st/120193.html (accessed October 29, 2014).
3. Heart and Vascular Institute, George Washington University, "Heart Facts," http://www.gwheartandvascular.org/media-center/heart-facts/ (accessed October 29, 2014).
4. Alan S. Go, Dariush Mozaffarian, Veronique L. Roger, et al., "Heart Disease and Stroke Statistics—2014 Update: A Report From the American Heart Association," *Circulation* 129, no. 3 (January 21, 2014): e28–e291, http://circ.ahajournals.org/content/129/3/e28.full.pdf+html (accessed October 29, 2014).
5. Million Hearts: The Initiative, US Department of Health and Human Services, "About Heart Disease and Stroke," http://millionhearts.hhs.gov/abouthds/cost-consequences.html (accessed October 29, 2014).

6. H. C. McGill Jr., C. A. McMahan, A. W. Zieske, et al., "Association of Coronary Heart Disease Risk Factors With Microscopic Qualities of Coronary Atherosclerosis in Youth," *Circulation* 102, no. 4 (July 25, 2000): 374–379.
7. William Davis, "New Blood Test Better Predicts Heart Attack Risk," *Life Extension*, May 2006, 60.
8. W. J. Elliott and L. H. Powell, "Diagonal Earlobe Creases and Prognosis in Patients With Suspected Coronary Artery Disease," *American Journal of Medicine* 100, no. 2 (February 1996): 205–211.
9. Dean Haycock, "Are Balding Men at Risk?" WebMD Feature, July 27, 2001, http://www.medicinenet.com/script/main/art.asp?articlekey=51027 (accessed October 29, 2014).
10. ScienceDaily.com, "More Fallout From Plaque Ruptures in Store for Heart Attack Survivors," July 23, 2002, http://www.sciencedaily.com/releases/2002/07/020724081223.htm (accessed October 29, 2014).
11. Davis, "New Blood Test Better Predicts Heart Attack Risk," 63.
12. Maria Cesarone, Andrea Di Renzo, Silvia Errichi, Frank Schonlau, James L. Wilmer, and Julian Blumenfield, "Improvement in Circulation and in Cardiovascular Risk Factors With a Proprietary Isotonic Bioflavonoid Formula OPC-3," *Journal of Angiology* 59, no. 4 (August/September 2008): 408–414.
13. American Heart Association, "Heart Disease and Stroke Continue to Threaten U.S. Health," December 18, 2013, http://newsroom.heart.org/news/heart-disease-and-stroke-continue-to-threaten-u-s-health (accessed October 29, 2014).

14. Donald Lloyd-Jones, Robert J. Adams, Todd M. Brown, et al., "Heart Disease and Stroke Statistics—2010 Update: A Report From the American Heart Association," *Circulation* 121, no. 7 (February 23, 2010): e46–e215; http://circ.ahajournals.org/content/121/7/e46.full (accessed October 29, 2014).

Chapter 2
Weight Gain

1. Centers for Disease Control and Prevention, "FastStats: Obesity and Overweight," http://www.cdc.gov/nchs/fastats/obesity-overweight.htm (accessed October 29, 2014).

2. Assistant Secretary for Planning and Evaluation, US Department of Health and Human Services, "Scope of the Problem: Overweight and Obesity," http://aspe.hhs.gov/health/blueprint/scope.shtml (accessed October 29, 2014).

3. Eric A. Finkelstein, Justin G. Trogdon, Joel W. Cohen, and William Dietz, "Annual Medical Spending Attributable to Obesity: Payer- and Service-Specific Estimates," *Health Affairs* 28, no. 5 (July 27, 2009): w822-w831; http://content.healthaffairs.org/content/28/5/w822.full.pdf+html (accessed October 29, 2014).

4. McDonalds.com, "Company Profile," http://www.aboutmcdonalds.com/mcd/investors/company_profile.html (accessed October 29, 2014); Index Mundi, "Country Comparison: Population," http://www.indexmundi.com/g/r.aspx (accessed October 29, 2014).

5. Alicia G. Walton, "How Much Sugar Are Americans Eating [Infographic]," Forbes.com, August 30, 2012, http://www.forbes.com/sites/alicegwalton/2012/08/30/how-much-sugar-are-americans-eating-infographic/ (accessed October 29, 2014).

6. William Davis, *Wheat Belly* (New York: Rodale, 2011), 14.

7. H. C. Broeck, H. C. de Jong, E. M. Salentijn, et al., "Presence of Celiac Disease Epitopes in Modern and Old Hexaploid Wheat Varieties: Wheat Breeding May Have Contributed to Increased Prevalence of Celiac Disease," *Theoretical and Applied Genetics* 121, no. 8 (November 2010): 1527–1539, as referenced in Davis, *Wheat Belly*, 26.

8. Davis, *Wheat Belly*, 35.

9. Ibid., 36, 53–54.

10. Ibid., 45.

11. ScienceDaily.com, "Obesity Increases Cancer Risk, Analysis of Hundreds of Studies Shows," February 18, 2008, http://www.sciencedaily.com/releases/2008/02/080217211802.htm (accessed October 29, 2014).

12. The Healthier Life.com, "GERD: Obesity Can Increase Your Risk of Acid Reflux Disease," March 29, 2006, http://www.thehealthierlife.co.uk/natural-health-articles/digestive-problems/gerd-obesity-increase-risk-00212.html (accessed October 29, 2014).

13. Frank Mangano, "The Obesity-Hypertension Connection: Your Weight May be Putting You at Risk," NaturalNews.com, July 27, 2009, http://www.naturalnews.com/026702_weight_blood_pressure.html (accessed October 29, 2014).

14. Krisha McCoy, "Your Body Fat Percentage: What Does It Mean?", NYU Langone Medical Center, December 18, 2012, http://www.med.nyu.edu/content?ChunkIID=41373 (accessed October 29, 2014).

15. Amanda Spake, "The Belly Burden," *U.S. News & World Report*, November 28, 2005, 72.

16. G. Davi, M. T. Guagnano, G. Ciabattoni, et al., "Platelet Activation in Obese Women: Role of Inflammation and Oxidant Stress," *Journal of the American Medical Association* 288, no. 16 (2002): 2008–2014.

17. B. B. Duncan, M. I. Schmidt, L. E. Chambless, A. R. Folsom, and G. Heiss, "Atherosclerosis Risk in Communities Study Investigators: Inflammation Markers Predict Increased Weight Gain in Smoking Quitters," *Obesity Research* 11, no. 11 (November 2003): 1339–1344; and E. Barinas-Mitchell, M. Cushman, E. N. Meilahn, R. P. Tracy, and L. H. Kuller, "Serum Levels of C-Reactive Protein Are Associated With Obesity, Weight Gain, and Hormone Replacement Therapy in Healthy Postmenopausal Women," *American Journal of Epidemiology* 153, no. 11 (June 2001): 1094–1101.

18. G. Engstrom, B. Hedblad, L. Stavenow, P. Lind, L. Janzon, and F. Lindgarde, "Inflammation-Sensitive Plasma Proteins Are Associated With Future Weight Gain," *Diabetes* 52, no. 8 (August 2003): 2097–2101.

19. Andrea Markowitz, "Forbidden Fruits and Other Foods," *Chicago Tribune*, July 26, 2010, http://articles.chicagotribune.com/2010-07-26/health/sc-health-0723-allergies-food-20100723_1_food-intolerance-food-allergies-anaphylactic-reaction (accessed October 30, 2014).

Chapter 3
Diabetes

1. Wikipedia, s.v. "Super Size Me," http://en.wikipedia.org/wiki/Supersize_me (accessed October 30, 2014).

2. Mary Clare Jalonick, "Obesity Rates Still Rising," *Huffington Post*, July 7, 2011, http://www.huffingtonpost.com/2011/07/07/obesity-states-rates_n_892181.html (accessed October 30, 2014).

3. Centers for Disease Control and Prevention, "Overweight and Obesity: Adult Obesity Facts," http://www.cdc.gov/obesity/data/adult.html (accessed October 30, 2014).

4. A. H. Mokdad, J. S. Marks, D. F. Stroup, and J. L. Gerberding, "Actual Causes of Death in the United States, 2000," *Journal of the American Medical Association* 291, no. 10 (March 10, 2004): 1238–1245.

5. Catherine Pearson, "Smoking Rates: Pack-A-Day Smoking Is Down Dramatically," *Huffington Post*, March 16, 2011, http://www.huffingtonpost.com/2011/03/16/smoking-rates-_n_835536.html (accessed October 30, 2014).

6. Associated Press, "Obesity Rates in U.S. Leveling Off," MSNBC.com, November 28, 2007, http://www.nbcnews.com/id/22007477/ns/health-diet_and_nutrition/t/obesity-rates-us-leveling#.VFI-UTTF_L8 (accessed October 30, 2014).

7. Centers for Disease Control and Prevention, "National Diabetes Fact Sheet, 2011" http://www.cdc.gov/diabetes/pubs/pdf/ndfs_2011.pdf (accessed October 30, 2014).

8. Ibid.

9. Gary Taubes, "Is Sugar Toxic?" *New York Times Magazine*, April 13, 2011, http://www.nytimes.com/2011/04/17/magazine/mag-17Sugar-t.html? (accessed October 30, 2014).

10. World Health Organization, "Diabetes," Fact Sheet N312, http://www.who.int/mediacentre/factsheets/fs312/en/ (accessed November 6, 2014).

11. Centers for Disease Control and Prevention, "National Diabetes Fact Sheet, 2011."

12. Ibid.

13. Ibid.

14. Centers for Disease Control and Prevention, "FastStats: Obesity and Overweight."

15. Michael Pollan, *In Defense of Food: An Eater's Manifesto* (New York: Penguin Press, 2008), 116.

16. Y. Wang, E. B. Rimm, M. J. Stampfer, W. C. Willet, and F. B. Hu, "Comparison of Abdominal Adiposity and Overall Obesity in Predicting Risk of Type 2 Diabetes Among Men," *American Journal of Clinical Nutrition* 81, no. 3 (March 2005): 555–563.

17. Eric Schlosser, *Fast Food Nation* (New York: Houghton Mifflin, 2001), 3, 242.

18. K. M. Venkat Narayan, James P. Boyle, Theodore J. Thompson, Stephen W. Sorensen, and David F. Williamson, "Lifetime Risk for Diabetes Mellitus in the United States," *Journal of the American Medical Association* 290, no. 14 (2003): 1884–1890.

19. United States Department of Health and Human Services, Office of the Surgeon General, "Overweight in Children and Adolescents," *The Surgeon General's Call to Action to Prevent and Decrease Overweight and Obesity*, viewed at West Virginia Department of Health and Human Resources, http://www.wvdhhr.org/bph/oehp/hp/obesity/fact_adolescents.htm (accessed October 30, 2014).

20. Centers for Disease Control and Prevention, "Adolescent and School Health: Childhood Obesity Facts," http://www.cdc.gov/healthyyouth/obesity/facts.htm (accessed October 30, 2014).

21. Michael F. Jacobson, *Liquid Candy: How Soft Drinks Are Harming Americans' Health* (Washington, DC: Center for Science in the Public Interest, 2005), 8–11.

22. MrBreakfast.com, "The Early Days of Breakfast Cereal," http://www.mrbreakfast.com/article.asp?articleid=13 (accessed October 30, 2014).

23. Rod Taylor, Carole Schmidt, and Lynn Kaladjian, "The Beanie Factor," *Brandweek*, June 16, 1997, abstract viewed at http://business.highbeam.com/137330/article-1G1-19505915/beanie-factor (accessed October 30, 2014).

24. Dan Morse, "School Cafeterias Are Enrolling as Fast-Food Franchises," *Wall Street Journal*, July 28, 1998, B2.

25. A. J. Stunkard, T. I. Sorensen, C. Hanis, et al., "An Adoption Study of Human Obesity," *New England Journal of Medicine* 314, no. 4 (1986): 193–198.

26. National Heart, Lung, and Blood Institute, National Institutes of Health, "What Causes Overweight and Obesity?" http://www.nhlbi.nih.gov/health/health-topics/topics/obe/causes.html (accessed October 30, 2014).

27. Pamela Peeke, *Fight Fat After Forty* (New York: Viking, 2000), 58.

28. Woodruff Health Sciences Center, "Excess Fat Puts Patients with Type 2 Diabetes at Greater Risk," news release, March 26, 2009, http://shared.web.emory.edu/whsc/news/releases/2009/03/excess-fat-puts-diabetic-patients-at-risk.html (accessed October 30, 2014).

29. Tamar Levin, "Record Level of Stress Found in College Freshmen," *New York Times*, January 26, 2011, http://www.nytimes.com/2011/01/27/education/27colleges.html (accessed November 2, 2011).

30. Centers for Disease Control and Prevention, "National Diabetes Fact Sheet, 2011."

31. American Diabetes Association, "Living With Diabetes: A1C and eAG," http://www.diabetes.org/

living-with-diabetes/treatment-and-care/blood-glucose-control/a1c/ (accessed October 30, 2014).

32. Centers for Disease Control and Prevention, "National Diabetes Fact Sheet, 2011."

33. Ibid.

34. National Diabetes Information Clearinghouse, "Diagnosis of Diabetes," http://diabetes.niddk.nih.gov/dm/pubs/diagnosis/ (accessed October 30, 2014).

35. Centers for Disease Control and Prevention, "National Diabetes Fact Sheet, 2011."

36. Ibid.

37. Ibid.

38. Ibid.

39. American Diabetes Association, "Diabetes Basics: Diabetes Symptoms," http://www.diabetes.org/diabetes-basics/symptoms/?loc=DropDownDB-symptoms (accessed October 30, 2014).

40. Ibid.

41. American Diabetes Association, "Epidemiology of Diabetes Interventions and Complications (EDIC): Design, Implementation, and Preliminary Results of a Long-Term Follow-Up of the Diabetes Control and Complications Trial Cohort," *Diabetes Care* 22, no. 1 (January 1999): 99–111, referenced in William Davis, *Wheat: The Unhealthy Whole Grain*, book excerpt "Wheat Belly," *Life Extension*, October 2011, http://www.lef.org/magazine/mag2011/oct2011_Wheat-The-Unhealthy-Whole-Grain_01.htm (accessed October 30, 2014).

42. Ibid.

43. K. T. Khaw, N. Wareham, R. Luben, et al., "Glycated Haemoglobin, Diabetes, and Mortality in Men in Norfolk Cohort of European Prospective Investigation of

Cancer and Nutrition (EPIC-Norfolk)," *British Medical Journal* 322, no. 7277 (January 6, 2001): 15–18, referenced in Davis, *Wheat: The Unhealthy Whole Grain*, book excerpt "Wheat Belly."

Chapter 4
Arthritis

1. National Institute of Arthritis and Musculoskeletal and Skin Diseases, National Institutes of Health, "Handout on Health: Osteoarthritis," August 2013, http://www.niams.nih.gov/Health_Info/Osteoarthritis/ (accessed October 30, 2014).
2. Centers for Disease Control and Prevention, "Arthritis: Osteoarthritis," May 2014, http://www.cdc.gov/arthritis/basics/osteoarthritis.htm (accessed October 30, 2014).
3. Centers for Disease Control and Prevention, "Arthritis: Rheumatoid Arthritis," November 19, 2012, http://www.cdc.gov/arthritis/basics/rheumatoid.htm (accessed November 3, 2014).
4. Eugene Braunwald, Anthony S. Fauci, Dennis L. Kasper, Stephen L. Hauser, Dan L. Longo, and J. Larry Jameson, ed., *Harrison's Principles of Internal Medicine*, 15th edition (New York: McGraw-Hill, 2001).
5. Rafael Ariza-Ariza, Marilu Mestanza-Peralta, and Mario H. Cardiel, "Omega-3 Fatty Acids in Rheumatoid Arthritis: An Overview," *Seminars in Arthritis and Rheumatism* 27, no. 6 (June 1998): 366–370.
6. Burton Goldberg Group, *Alternative Medicine: The Definitive Guide* (Puyallup, WA: Fullness Medicine Publishing, Inc., 1993), 532.
7. You can read more about this therapy in Devi S. Nambudripad's book *Say Good-bye to Illness*, 3rd edition

(n.p.: Delta Publishers, 2002). You can also learn more at www.naet.com.

8. Ariza-Ariza, Mestanza-Peralta, and Cardiel, "Omega-3 Fatty Acids in Rheumatoid Arthritis: An Overview."
9. Selene Yeager and the editors of *Prevention*, *New Foods for Healing* (Emmaus, PA: Rodale Press, 1999), 171.
10. A. L Vaz, "Double-Blind Clinical Evaluation of the Relative Efficacy of Ibuprofen and Glucosamine Sulfate in the Management of Osteoarthritis of the Knee in Outpatients," *Current Medical Research and Opinion* 8 (1982): 145–149.
11. E. D. D'Ambrosio, B. Casa, R. Bompani, G. Scali, and M. Scali, "Glucosamine Sulfate: A Controlled Clinical Investigation in Arthrosis," *Pharmatherapeutica* 2 (1982): 504–508.

Chapter 5
How Metabolism Works

1. Meghan J. Ward, "Time Lapse Photography: Interview With John Novotny," *The Campsite* (blog), April 17, 2011, http://thecampsiteblog.com/2011/04/17/time-lapse-photography/ (accessed November 3, 2014).
2. Barbara Bushman and Janice Clark-Young, *Action Plan for Menopause* (Champaign, IL: American College of Sports Medicine, 2005), 68–70.
3. Ibid.
4. *Webster's New World College Dictionary*, 4th ed. (n.p.: Wiley Publishing, Inc., 2004), s.v. "metabolism."
5. Jim Harvey, "Measuring BMR in the Pulmonary Lab," *FOCUS: Journal for Respiratory Care and Sleep Medicine*, July 1, 2006, http://www.thefreelibrary.com/

Measuring+BMR+in+the+Pulmonary+lab.-a0186218061 (accessed November 4, 2014).

6. Osama Hamdy, Gabriel I. Uwaifo, and Elif A. Oral, "Obesity," Medscape.com, September 16, 2014, http://emedicine.medscape.com/article/123702-overview (accessed November 4, 2014).
7. J. A. Levine, L. M. Lanningham-Foster, S. K. McCrady, et al., "Interindividual Variation in Posture Allocation: Possible Role in Human Obesity," *Science* 307, no. 5709 (January 28, 2005): 584–586.
8. Lawrence C. Wood, David S. Cooper, and E. Chester Ridgeway, *Your Thyroid: A Home Reference* (New York: Ballantine Books, 1995).
9. H. K. Shames and E. Q. Youngkin, "The Thyroid Dance: Nursing Approaches to Autoimmune Low Thyroid," *AWHONN Lifelines* 6, no 1 (February–March 2002): 52–59.

Chapter 6
The Starch and Sugar Trap

1. H. Du, D. L. van der A, M. M. van Bakel, et al., "Glycemic Index and Glycemic Load in Relation to Food and Nutrient Intake and Metabolic Risk Factors in a Dutch Population," *American Journal of Clinical Nutrition* 87, no. 3 (March 2008): 655–661.
2. BestDietTips.com, "Glycemic Index List of Foods," http://www.bestdiettips.com/content/view/219/53/ (accessed December 26, 2014).
3. George A. Bray, Samara Joy Nielsen, and Barry M. Popkin, "Consumption of High-Fructose Corn Syrup in Beverages May Play a Role in the Epidemic of Obesity," *American Journal of Clinical Nutrition* 79, no. 4 (April 2004): 537–543.

Chapter 7
Right Knowledge for Eating Right

1. US Department of Health and Human Services, *Dietary Guidelines for Americans, 2010*, 7th ed. (Washington, DC: US Government Printing Office, 2010), 15; http://health.gov/dietaryguidelines/dga2010/DietaryGuidelines2010.pdf (accessed November 4, 2014).
2. M. Conceicao de Oliveira, R. Sichieri, and Moura A. Sanchez, "Weight Loss Associated With a Daily Intake of Three Apples or Three Pears Among Overweight Women," *Nutrition* 19, no. 3 (2003): 253–256.
3. Jack Challem, *The Inflammation Syndrome* (Hoboken, NJ: John Wiley & Sons, Inc., 2003).
4. Nancy C. Howarth, Terry T.-K. Huang, Susan B. Roberts, and Megan A. McCrory, "Dietary Fiber and Fat Are Associated With Excess Weight in Young and Middle-Aged US Adults," *Journal of the American Dietetic Association* 105, no. 9 (September 2005): 1365–1372.
5. Kate Murphy, "The Dark Side of Soy," BusinessWeek.com, December 18, 2000, http://www.businessweek.com/2000/00_51/b3712218.htm (accessed November 4, 2014).
6. R. Anand and P. Basiotis, "Is Total Fat Consumption Really Decreasing?" *Nutrition Insights* 5 (April 1998): http://www.cnpp.usda.gov/sites/default/files/nutrition_insights_uploads/insight5.pdf (accessed November 4, 2014).
7. Crisco.com, "Our History," http://www.crisco.com/About_Crisco/History.aspx (accessed November 4, 2014).
8. Associated Press, "Crisco Drops Trans Fat From Shortening Formula," MSNBC.com, January 25, 2007, http://www.msnbc.msn.com/id/16795455/ns/

health-diet_and_nutrition/t/crisco-drops-trans-fats -shortening-formula/ (accessed November 4, 2014).

9. Jane E. Brody, "Women's Heart Risk Linked to Types of Fats, Not Total," *New York Times*, November 20, 1997, http://www.nytimes.com/1997/11/20/us/women-s-heart -risk-linked-to-types-of-fats-not-total.html (accessed November 4, 2014).
10. Wendy DeMark-Wahnefried, ABC News, "A Donut for Your Diet? The Truth About Trans Fat," August 28, 2007, http://abcnews.go.com/Health/Diet/story?id=3121351 (accessed November 4, 2014).
11. Electronic Code of Federal Regulations, "Title 21: Food and Drugs, Section 101.9 Nutrition Labeling of Food," http://www.accessdata.fda.gov/scripts/cdrh/cfdocs/cfCFR/CFRSearch.cfm?fr=101.9 (accessed November 5, 2014).
12. American Heart Association, "Know Your Fats," July 31, 2014, http://www.heart.org/HEARTORG/Conditions/Cholesterol/PreventionTreatmentofHighCholesterol/Know-Your-Fats_UCM_305628_Article.jsp (accessed November 5, 2014).
13. Anthony Kane, "Omega-3 Fatty Acids and Depression," ADDADHDAdvances.com, http://addadhdadvances .com/efa-depression.html (accessed November 5, 2014).
14. Ancel Keys, *Seven Countries: A Multivariate Analysis of Death and Coronary Heart Disease* (Boston: Harvard University Press, 1980).
15. As referenced in Elizabeth Somer, "Should I Consume Olive Oil if I'm Trying to Lose Weight?", April 30, 2001, http://greekfamilyoil.weebly.com/should-i-consume -olive-oil-if-im-trying-to-lose-weight.html (accessed November 5, 2014).

Chapter 8
Beating Inflammation the Natural Way

1. Clara Felix, *All About Omega-3 Oils* (Garden City, NY: Avery Publishing, 1998), 32.
2. MedicalNewsToday.com, "Mediterranean-Style Diet Reduces Cancer and Heart Disease Risk," June 26, 2003, http://www.medicalnewstoday.com/articles/3835.php (accessed November 5, 2014).
3. Antonia Trichopoulou, Pagona Lagiou, Hannah Kupeer, and Dimitrios Trichopoulos, "Cancer and the Mediterranean Dietary Traditions," *Cancer Epidemiology, Biomarkers and Prevention* 9 (September 2009): 869–873.
4. "Mercury Contamination in Fish: A Guide to Staying Healthy and Fighting Back," Natural Resources Defense Council, http://www.nrdc.org/health/effects/mercury/guide.asp (accessed November 5, 2014).
5. L. S. Gross, L. Li, E. S. Ford, and S. Liu, "Increased Consumption of Refined Carbohydrates and the Epidemic of Type 2 Diabetes in the United States: An Ecological Assessment," *American Journal of Clinical Nutrition* 79, no. 5 (2004): 774–779.
6. Ibid.
7. Marian Burros, "Stores Say Wild Salmon, but Tests Say Farm Bred," *New York Times*, April 10, 2005, http://www.nytimes.com/2005/04/10/dining/10salmon.html?scp=1&sq=stores+say+wild+salmon&st=nyt (accessed November 5, 2014).
8. Lauren Muney, "Top 10 Excuses for Falling off the Diet/Fitness Wagon—and Answer for Them," PhysicalMind.com, http://www.physicalmind.com/articles.html (accessed November 7, 2011). No longer available online.

9. Robert Preidt, "Mom Was Right: Eating Soup Cuts Calorie Intake," May 1, 2007, ABCNews.com, http://abcnews.go.com/Health/Healthday/story?id=4506787 (accessed November 5, 2014).

10. ScienceDaily.com, "Teens Who Eat Breakfast Daily Eat Healthier Diets Than Those Who Skip Breakfast," March 3, 2008, http://www.sciencedaily.com/releases/2008/03/080303072640.htm (accessed November 5, 2014).

11. Jennie Brand-Miller, Thomas M. S. Wolever, Kaye Foster-Powell, and Stephen Colagiuri, *The New Glucose Revolution*, 3rd ed., (New York: Marlow & Co., 2007), 86.

12. National Restaurant Association, "Restaurant Industry Sales Turn Positive in 2011 After Three Tough Years," RestaurantNews.com, February 1, 2011, http://www.restaurantnews.com/restaurant-industry-sales-turn-positive-in-2011-after-three-tough-years/ (accessed November 5, 2014).

13. David Zinczenko with Matt Goulding, *Eat This, Not That!* (New York: Rodale Books, 2008), 113.

Chapter 9
Get Your Exercise Groove On

1. Caroline J. Cedarquist, "Fitness With Fido: A Healthy Pastime for Dog Owners," *Sandoval Signpost*, February 2006, http://www.sandovalsignpost.com/feb06/html/animal_hotline.html (accessed November 5, 2014).

2. Levine, Lanningham-Foster, McCrady, et al., "Interindividual Variation in Posture Allocation: Possible Role in Human Obesity."

3. K. Boutelle and D. Kirschenbaum, "Further Support for Consistent Self-Monitoring as a Vital Component of

Successful Weight Control," *Obesity Research* 6, no. 3 (May 1998): 219–224.

4. Peter Jaret, "A Healthy Mix of Rest and Motion," *New York Times*, May 3, 2007, http://tinyurl.com/c7zxot3 (accessed November 5, 2014).
5. Centers for Disease Control and Prevention, "How Much Physical Activity Do Adults Need?", December 1, 2011, http://www.cdc.gov/physicalactivity/everyone/guidelines/adults.html (accessed November 5, 2014).

Chapter 10
Support It With Supplements

1. Michael Johnson, "Obesity Epidemic Feeds Weight-Loss Product Sales," DrugStoreNews.com, January 5, 2011, http://www.drugstorenews.com/article/obesity-epidemic-feeds-weight-loss-product-sales (accessed November 5, 2014).
2. P. Chantre and D. Lairon, "Recent Findings of Green Tea Extract AR25 (Exolise) and Its Activity for the Treatment of Obesity," *Phytomedicine* 9, no. 1 (January 2002): 3–8.
3. LifeExtension.org, "Abstracts: Green Coffee Bean Extract," *Life Extension Magazine*, February 2012, http://www.lef.org/Magazine/2012/2/Magnesium-L-Threonate-UC-II-Metformin-Green-Coffee-Bean-Extract-and-Postprandial-Glucose-Levels/Page-04 (accessed November 5, 2014).
4. Douglas Laboratories, "Metabolic Management Pack: Nutritional Support for Healthy Weight Management," product data sheet, June 2012, http://www.douglaslabs.com/media/DL66212.pdf (accessed November 5, 2014).

5. American Thyroid Association, "Iodine Deficiency," June 4, 2012, http://www.thyroid.org/iodine-deficiency/ (accessed November 5, 2014).
6. J. A. Marlett, M. I. McBurney, J. L. Slavin, and American Dietetic Association, "Position of the American Dietetic Association: Health Implications of Dietary Fiber," *Journal of the American Dietetic Association* 102, no. 7 (2002): 993–1000.
7. N. C. Howarth, E. Saltzman, and S. B. Roberts, "Dietary Fiber and Weight Regulation," *Nutrition Review* 59, no. 5 (2001): 129–138.
8. Lisa E. Bolton, Americus Reed II, Kevin G. Volpp, and Katrina Armstrong, "How Does Drug and Supplement Marketing Affect a Healthy Lifestyle?", *Journal of Consumer Research* 34 (February 2008).
9. Andrew Weil, "7-Keto: Supplement to Speed Metabolism?" DrWeil.com, http://www.drweil.com/drw/u/QAA401158/7Keto-Supplement-to-Speed-Metabolism.html (accessed November 5, 2014).
10. "7-Keto-DHEA," WebMD.com, http://tinyurl.com/7okmz6n (accessed November 5, 2014).
11. Weil, "7-Keto: Supplement to Speed Metabolism?"
12. J. L. Zenk, J. L. Frestedt, and M. A. Kuskowski, "HUM5007, a Novel Combination of Thermogenic Compounds, and 3-Acetyl-7-Oxo-Dehydroepiandrosterone: Each Increases the Resting Metabolic Rate of Overweight Adults," *Journal of Nutritional Biochemistry* 18, no. 9 (September 2007): 629–634; and Michael Davidson, Ashok Marwah, Ronald J. Sawchuk, et. al., "Safety and Pharmacokinetic Study With Escalating Doses of 3-Acetyl-7-Oxo-Dehydroepiandrosterone in Healthy Male Volunteers," *Clinical Investigative Medicine* 23, no. 5 (October 2000): 300–310.

13. Hoodia Advice, "The Science of Hoodia," http://www.hoodia-advice.org/hoodia-plant.html (accessed November 5, 2014).
14. Tom Mangold, "Sampling the Kalahari Hoodia Diet," BBC News, May 30, 2003, http://news.bbc.co.uk/2/hi/programmes/correspondent/2947810.stm (accessed November 5, 2014).
15. Ano Lobb, "Hepatoxicity Associated With Weight-Loss Supplements: A Case for Better Post-Marketing Surveillance," *World Journal of Gastroenterology* 15, no. 14 (April 14, 2009): 1786–1787.
16. Associated Press, "FDA Warns Consumers to Avoid Brazilian Diet Pills," USAToday.com, January 13, 2006, http://usatoday30.usatoday.com/news/health/2006-01-13-brazilian-diet-pills_x.htm (accessed March 26, 2013).

INDEX

D

E

F

G

H

O

P

R

S

T

U

V

W

Y